Stress-induced Analgesia

Stress-induced Analgesia

Edited by

M. D. TRICKLEBANK
Merrell-Dow, Research Center
Strasbourg

and

G. CURZON
Institute of Neurology,
University of London

A Wiley–Interscience Publication

JOHN WILEY & SONS
Chichester · New York · Brisbane · Singapore · Toronto

Library of Congress Cataloging in Publication Data:
Main entry under title:

Stress-induced analgesia.

'A Wiley–Interscience publication.'
Based on a workshop held at a meeting in Jerusalem of the
Collegium Internationale Nuero-Psychopharmacologicum, 1982.
Includes index.
1. Pain—Prevention—Congresses. 2. Analgesia—
Congresses. 3. Stress (Physiology)—Congresses.
4. Counter-irritants—Congresses. I. Tricklebank, M. D.
II. Curzon, G. (Gerald), 1928– . [DNLM: 1. Pain—
Physiopathology—Congresses. 2. Stress—Physiopathology
—Congresses. WL 704 S915 1982]
OP451.4.S77 1984 612′.88 84-5265

ISBN 0 471 90430 9

British Library Cataloguing in Publication Data:

Stress-induced analgesia.
1. Pain 2. Analgesia 3. Stress (Psychology)
4. Stress (Physiology)
I. Tricklebank, M.D. II. Curzon, G.
616′.0472 RB127

ISBN 0 471 90430 9

Typeset by Activity Ltd, Salisbury, Wilts.
Printed by Pitman Press Ltd, Bath, Avon

Contributors

H. Anisman
Department of Psychology, Carleton University, Ottawa, Canada

T. Archer
Department of Pharmacology, Research and Development Laboratories, Astra Lakemedel AB, S–151 85, Sodertalje, Sweden

R. J. Bodnar
Department of Psychology, Queens College, City University of New York, Flushing, New York 11367, USA

S. Cadden
Unité de Recherches de Neurophysiologie Pharmacologique, INSERM (U.161), 2 rue d'Alésia, 75014, Paris, France

B. Calvino
Unité de Recherches de Neurophysiologie Pharmacologique, INSERM (U.161), 2 rue d'Alésia, 75014, Paris, France

G. Curzon
Department of Neurochemistry, Institute of Neurology, 33 John's Mews, London WC1N 2NS, UK

M. Devor
Life Sciences Institute, Hebrew University of Jerusalem, Jerusalem 91904, Israel

P. H. Hutson
Department of Neurochemistry, Institute of Neurology, 33 John's Mews, London WC1N 2NS, UK

C. Johansson
Department of Pharmacology, Research and Development Laboratories, Astra Lakemedel AB, S-151 85, Sodertalje, Sweden

D. Le Bars
Unité de Recherches de Neurophysiologie Pharmacologique, INSERM (U.161), 2 rue d'Alésia, 75014, Paris, France

J. W. Lewis
Department of Psychology, University of California, Los Angeles, California 90024, USA

J. C. Liebeskind
Department of Psychology, University of California, Los Angeles, California 90024, USA

L. R. Nelson
Department of Psychology, University of California, Los Angeles, California 90024, USA

S. -O. Ogren
Department of Pharmacology, Research and Development Laboratories, Astra Lakemedel AB, S–151 85, Sodertalje, Sweden

G. W. Terman
Department of Psychology, University of California, Los Angeles, California 90024, USA

M. D. Tricklebank
Merrell-Dow Research Center, 16 rue d'Ankara, 67084, Strasbourg Cedex, France

L. Villanueva
Unité de Recherches de Neurophysiologie Pharmacologique, INSERM (U.161), 2 rue d'Alésia, 75014, Paris, France

R. M. Zacharko
Department of Psychology, Carleton University, Ottawa, Canada

Contents

Preface

Familiar stories such as that of the wartime pilot successfully landing his plane apparently oblivious of his injuries, vividly illustrate the power of endogenous analgesia mechanisms. The awareness since ancient times that purposely inflicted pain can control pain of pathological origin is indicated by the Latin proverb 'pro medicina est dolor dolorem qui necat' (the pain that kills pain acts as medicine). However, it is only with the advent of modern behavioural, electrophysiological, pharmacological, and neurochemical techniques that we have begun to understand endogenous pain inhibitory systems. The following chapters indicate the remarkable amount of progress that has recently been made.

Research into stress-induced analgesia has relevance to numerous topics: to anaesthesia, acupuncture and placebo reactions, to the mechanisms by which stress affects behaviour and to such related phenomena as learned helplessness and other animal models of depression. It is an attractive field to the investigator, not least because methods by which stress-induced analgesia can be produced provide remarkably simple and reliable means of studying neurochemical and pharmacological aspects of pain control. They are thus powerful laboratory tools for elucidating nociceptive processes and the improved understanding that should be obtained by their use may lead to new methods for the alleviation of pain.

This volume derives from a workshop held during the recent meeting at Jerusalem of the Collegium Internationale Neuro-Psychopharmacologicum. We thank Astra Lakemedel AB for financial support of the workshop and Dr S. O. Ogren for his help in arranging this support.

M. D. Tricklebank
G. Curzon

Stress-induced Analgesia
Edited by M. D. Tricklebank and G. Curzon

CHAPTER 1

Pain and 'state'-induced analgesia: an introduction

M. DEVOR

According to the Subcommittee on Taxonomy of the International Association for the Study of Pain (IASP), pain is 'an unpleasant sensory and emotional experience associated with actual or potential tissue damage, or described in terms of such damage' (see *Pain*, **6** (1979), 250). This definition clearly distinguishes the pain under examination from, say, the 'pain' (grief) of losing a loved one, the 'pain' (disappointment) of unfulfilled expectation, or the 'pain' (exasperation) of attending an interminable meeting. It also clearly recognizes that pain can and frequently does arise in the absence of noxious (tissue threatening) stimuli, and points to a way of understanding such pains. All things being normal, a burn on the hand activates a specific subset of central nerve cells and the activity of this cell assembly constitutes the pain (Hebb, 1949). If the same central cell assembly were similarly activated in the same way by some other means, for example by abnormal discharge originating in a region of nerve damage, or by spontaneous 'epileptic' activity, the experience would be the same, that is, burning pain in the hand. Analgesia is quite simply a reduction in the activity of the pain assembly.

In principle, it should be possible to produce analgesia at will by blocking conduction pathways that excite the pain assembly, or by depressing neural activity either at the level of the impulse generator or in the pain assembly itself. In the peripheral nervous system, where neural circuitry is relatively spread out, artificial conduction block and pharmacological inhibition is often practical. However, when it comes to the central nervous system (CNS) with its intricate compactness, the techniques available to us are far too crude and clumsy to be really effective.

There is, however, another approach. Ever since Sherrington (1906), it has been appreciated that neural mechanisms generally involve both excitation and inhibition and abundant evidence collected over several decades indicates that central pain mechanisms are no exception. If one could selectively tap into an already existing inhibitory system, then effective control of activity in the central pain assembly should be possible.

As often occurs, hints of how this might be accomplished are provided by folk medicine and traditional pain management practices. One such hint is the effectiveness of naturally occurring medicinal agents. Systematic study of the mechanisms of action of extracts of the opium poppy (*Papaver somniferum*), for example, may lead to dramatic improvements in the effectiveness and reliability of opiate drugs. Another traditional approach to the relief of pain, one that is also presumably based on tapping into endogenous pain control circuitry, is the induction of special emotional 'states' in the sufferer. There is little doubt that under the right conditions the soothing sound of a mother's voice, or needle pricks administered by a famous healer can be very powerful medicine indeed. True, these 'psychological' effects are not very reliable even under ideal conditions, and in the hands of experienced practitioners. Even the most credulous must doubt whether such 'medicine' could ever be mass produced and supplied in 100 ml injection vials. None the less, this should not obscure the central point that powerful endogenous pain control mechanisms exist and are subject to artificial access.

In this chapter I will begin by discussing some of the inherent limitations of attempts to block central pain pathways or suppress impulse generators. Then I will consider endogenous pain control mechanisms, with respect to both their evolution and to some of the general properties of the relevant central neural circuits. Finally, I will ask how one might be able to engage these circuits by artificial means.

BLOCKING IMPULSES

Like a rumour passing through a crowd, there are a lot of places at which a pain message might be stopped, but few whose blockade will prevent the message from eventually getting through. To achieve analgesia by means of conduction block or focal suppression, one tries to identify nodal points in the network. Sometimes, for example, it is possible to identify a localized source of the nerve impulses and to prevent their initiation. If the source were an actual stimulus like heat, the stimulus could be excluded, or the impulse generator (e.g. thermo-sensitive afferent endings in the skin) could be deadened. Sometimes sensory endings originally specialized to report on noxious events become abnormally sensitive and discharge in response to normally innocuous stimuli. Ideally, the hypersensitivity should be reversible. A similar situation arises when impulses are generated at a site of nerve injury and here too it may be possible to reverse the changes which lead to ectopic impulse generation (Devor and Govrin-Lippmann, 1983).

In circumstances in which the generator of offending impulses is diffused, or for some other reason cannot be attacked directly, it may still be possible to block the forward conduction of the discharge. This might be done by blocking peripheral nerve or brain tract conduction, or by blocking information transfer across intervening synapses. The problem here is that very shortly after entry into the spinal cord the transmission of 'pain' signals, like the spread of rumours, tends to become multiplexed, with some of the channels being highly diffuse and polysynaptic. For this reason anterolateral cordotomy and transection of other compact central fibre tracts is notoriously ineffective in producing long-term pain relief in animals or man.

Finally, one could ignore the generators and the conductors and try to selectively anaesthetize the central pain assembly itself. Given our present state of knowledge, however, this is the most difficult approach of all. In fact, it may not be possible even in principle. There are two reasons for this. Firstly, it is highly unlikely that the pain assembly is located in one confined area. It is more likely to be diffused in a widespread network throughout the brain and dependent on many different functional modes and neurotransmitters. Secondly, individual cells involved in pain perception are probably also involved in other important functions as well, and it may be impossible to block their contribution to one system without disrupting others at the same time. This dilemma is at the heart of the concept of the 'grandmother assembly', a hypothetical set of central visual cells whose net activity defines the experience of seeing grandmother in the same way that our 'pain assembly' defines the experience of pain. Jerome Lettvin, from whom I first heard this account, asks what would happen if with consummate surgical skill one were to kill off all of the cells in the 'grandmother assembly' without harming any others. By definition, grandmother is no longer recognized. But then, he continues, who is that lady who lives at 225 Markham Street and who sleeps with grandfather (note that cells of the 'grandfather assembly' have not been eliminated) and who makes such unforgettable chicken soup? And so, grandmother has returned! Obviously, if all the cells whose activity is linked to grandmother were eliminated, the deficit would extend well beyond grandmother herself, perhaps most of the way to unconsciousness.

The problems of distribution and multiplexing do not, however, mean that to say 'pain assembly' is the same as to say 'the brain'. There are obviously some major brain structures and functions that are so distantly related to pain as to be clearly excludable. It is probably safe to include in these, the ventral grey of the spinal cord, the cerebellum, pons, much of the thalamus, the basal ganglia, etc. One surprising, but so far consistent finding is the lack of an obvious pain representation in the somatosensory cortex, or any other part of the cerebral convexity (Penfield and Rasmussen, 1950; Semmes, 1973). However, these cortical areas obviously respond to pain, as we can talk about it, and they are clearly involved in memory about pain, behavioural strategies concerning pain and cognitive reflections about its significance. What then are the likely limits within which the central pain assembly and its attendant inhibitory network lie?

Structurally, we are probably talking about a web of cells scattered throughout the dorsal and intermediate grey of the spinal cord including corresponding spinal trigeminal structures, the brainstem reticular formation, certain parts of the thalamus, much of the limbic system including Nauta's limbic midbrain circuit (Nauta, 1958) and mesial temporal and orbital limbic cortex. Essentially, we are talking about what goes on after sensory transduction and coding, and before the systems that organize action on the one hand, and concept and memory formation on the other.

FUNCTION OF ENDOGENOUS PAIN CONTROL

Pain serves to warn us of situations in which mechanical, thermal, or chemical stimuli are dangerously strong, and it is thus a fundamentally desirable (adaptive) thing. Indeed, individuals without it are seriously handicapped (Brand, 1973; Sweet, 1981). It is therefore not surprising that the pain system like other highly adaptive biological mechanisms, has dynamic controls built-in to modify its operation as need dictates. For example, there are times when fairly weak stimuli can injure tissue (e.g. on sunburned skin or over a scrape) and extra protection is called for. Under such circumstances some classes of cutaneous nociceptive afferents become 'sensitized' so that they signal pain at appropriately reduced levels of stimulus intensity. There are other times when there is no escape from the noxious stimulus, or when such escape is simply too expensive in terms of other goals of the organism. These situations may have forced the evolution of internal mechanisms which decrease pain.

Escape from noxious stimuli is among the most primaeval of sensory-motor phenomena. Even the most primitive single-celled organisms that are capable of independent movement (bacteria) can link the direction of their movement to gradients of noxious influences (negative chemotaxis, thermotaxis, etc.). This essentially automatic capability, which in its simplest form obviously does not even require a nervous system, occurs in advanced vertebrates as the 'withdrawal' or 'flexor' reflexes. However, when there are both life-threatening and life-sustaining factors in the immediate environment, automatic withdrawal dictated at the level of the peripheral receptor or the first central synapse is no longer satisfactory. It becomes necessary to balance the danger against the advantage; a 'decision' must be made. The need for higher level, and ultimately cerebral control becomes even greater when the danger is immediate and the advantage lies somewhere in the future. Consider a lion attacking its prey, but being kicked by it before the kill is made. Or consider a buck defending its territory and harem against the potentially deadly antlers of a rival. Or consider the rival. In these situations it is imperative for survival that higher cerebral processes are able to inhibit lower level reflexes and other antecedents of escape.

The design of neural circuitry capable of suppressing the tendency to escape in the face of noxious stimuli does not necessarily require that the experience of pain be suppressed as well. Because of its very nature and function, however, pain focuses attention and therefore tends to impair performance in other spheres. It seems intuitively obvious that natural selection would favour individuals who can process information in all realms at maximum efficiency during emergencies, and that those whose capacity is seriously degraded would not be able to compete. Observers of animals in the wild frequently describe apparent suppression of pain responses during crises. For example, Kruuk (1964) reports that hedgehogs gorging on eggs and chicks after successfully raiding a gull nest, appear (despite injury) to ignore swooping attacks made by the parent gulls. At early stages in the raid, such attacks induce retreat. Similarly, many species of lizards apparently painlessly abandon a fully innervated tail while escaping a pursuing predator. 'Playing dead' (death feigning), an anti-predator strategy used by a variety of species throughout the animal kingdom, may be an ultimate extension of environmentally triggered analgesic 'states'. For example, ducks otherwise totally alert suppress responses to mutilating injury, while awaiting an opportunity to escape (Ratner, 1967; Sargent and Eberhardt, 1975).

Spontaneous analgesia is also known to occur in man during crises. At times of grave danger, on the battlefield in war, for example, severe mutilating injuries are sometimes not felt as painful (Beecher, 1956). Many an anecdote describes the soldier dragging his buddy to safety, or fending off a last attack, only later to discover the cause of the warm, wet sensation on his leg. This is not a matter of heroic stoicism; there simply is no pain. Within a few hours, however, the pain invariably comes on, and like the rest of us, the soldier may well flinch and complain when on the next day a nurse is a bit too rough with the pin-prick of an injection.

ENDOGENOUS PAIN CONTROL MECHANISMS

The brain's ability to control the forward transmission of pain signals is probably expressed at each level of the pain network. However, for reasons that are partly historical and partly practical, the bulk of current research has concentrated on the long descending control pathways with final actions at the level of the spinal cord. Descending controls on spinal nociceptive reflexes have been well known at least since Sherington (1906). Credit for bringing to the fore the significance of these controls for pain perception, however, belongs to Melzack and Wall (1965) with their 'gate control theory' of pain. In 1965 it was not known whether descending pain control is mediated by specific, well delineated pathways, or as part of the diffuse and still rather mysterious 'descending reticular formation'. In the past 15 years both types of mechanism have been clearly implicated. In particular, as a result of a series of very clever experiments, much detailed information has accumulated on certain well defined spinal pathways descending from the brain stem (for reviews, see Basbaum and Fields, 1978; Fields and Basbaum, 1978; Gebhart, 1982; and Watkins and Mayer, 1982 among others). Here, I shall summarize only very briefly the current state of affairs. It is convenient to refer to three general groups of descending spinal controls:

(i) Long opiate-related systems.
(ii) Long non-opiate-related systems.
(iii) Diffuse inhibitory control systems.

Long opiate-related descending controls

This first group is certainly the best described today. It occurs in the caudal part of Nauta's limbic midbrain circuit: the ventral part of the periaqueductal grey matter and adjacent tegmentum, and the caudal walls of the third ventricle. Cells in this region are rich in opiate receptors and their activation by direct electrical stimulation or by local application of their putative natural transmitter group, the endogenous opioid peptides (enkephalins, endorphins, and dynorphin) produces a profound analgesia, without corresponding general behavioural depression. Severing the dorsolateral spinal white matter (the dorsolateral funiculus) largely blocks this analgesia ipsilaterally below the level of the cut. The influence of the periaqueductal grey at spinal levels is not, however, mediated by a direct descending pathway although direct mesencephalo-spinal and even hypothalamo-spinal fibres are known to exist. It acts rather via intermediate relay cells in the medulla. Two main relay nuclei have so far been identified, and others are implicated as well. One, the nucleus raphé magnus, is rich in serotonin and its action at the spinal level is presumably mediated largely by this neurotransmitter. The second is the nucleus reticularis magnocellularis whose neurotransmitter(s) is not yet known. A curious feature of the descending periaqueductal grey system is that it has at least two opiate related links. The most sensitive is in this system itself and indeed, it is believed that systemic opiates produce analgesia by acting here and exciting the descending pathway. The second link is in the dorsal horn of the spinal cord and particularly the substantia gelatinosa, where application of relatively high concentrations of opiates can produce local analgesia. There is evidence of synergism between spinal and supra spinal sites (Levine, *et al.*, 1982). The spinal opiate receptors are mainly on small diameter (nociceptor?) primary afferent terminals and their endogenous presynaptic elements are presumably local opiate-containing interneurones. The intricacies of the spinal synaptic relations of descending serotonin and non-serotonin containing fibres are the subject of much current research. It should be kept in mind that opiate receptors occur not only in the periaqueductal grey and the substantia gelatinosa, but are also widely distributed throughout the neuraxis (e.g. Herkenham and Pert, 1982). Despite the impressive progress that has been made, there clearly remains a great deal more to be learned about central opiate-related pathways.

Long non-opiate related pathways

The discovery of the powerful antinociceptive pathway descending from the periaqueductal grey to the substantia gelatinosa via the medulla has tended to promote the attitude that all intrinsic pain control phenomena operate by the release of endogenous opioids in the periaqueductal grey. This is plainly inaccurate. In fact, it became clear fairly early on that the analgesia produced by stimulation here is not fully blocked by opiate antagonists (e.g. naloxone) or by severing the dorsolateral funiculus (Basbaum *et al.*, 1977; Carstens *et al.*, 1979). This presumably means that there are long descending anti-nociceptive mechanisms originating in the periaqueductal grey that do not have an obligatory opiate relay and do not involve the dorsolateral funiculus. Furthermore, stimulation of many mesencephalic and rhombencephalic sites other than the periaqueductal grey produces descending inhibition. One such site is the locus coeruleus–subcoeruleus complex which sends descending nor-adrenaline-containing fibres via the funiculus directly to the substantia gelatinosa without an intervening synapse. For other such sites the course of the descending anti-nociceptive fibres remains to be worked out in detail. The elucidation of some non-funicular pathways may prove to be technically quite challenging. If such fibres travelled in either the dorsal, ventral, or anterolateral columns of the spinal cord for example, motor and/or sensory losses due to the transection of ascending fibres would probably complicate behavioural analysis, and antidromic activation would probably complicate electrophysiological analysis.

In addition to brainstem structures, many forebrain structures have long been implicated in descending spinal inhibition (Hagbarth and Kerr, 1954) and it is certainly premature to conclude that these inhibitions must all be mediated by the brainstem pathways already identified. For example, hypothalamic stimulation (and sometimes lesions) can produce a contralateral somatosensory 'neglect' syndrome that includes hypoalgesia. Similarly, electrical stimulation in many diencephalic and cortical loci (e.g. Wyon-Maillard *et al.*, 1972; Carstens *et al.*, 1982) can inhibit the discharge of spinal neurones including those with wide dynamic range (lamina 5-type) somatosensory input. Even the corticospinal (pyramidal) tract is thus implicated. Although generally considered a motor pathway, it has long been known that many, and in some species most, of its synaptic relations are with cells in the dorsal horn, and that many of its effects are inhibitory (Fetz, 1968; Pretel *et al.*, 1982).

Diffuse inhibitory control systems

The third group of descending controls remains in the sphere of the descending reticular formation and involve a slowly conducting, polysynaptic, only crudely topographic (diffuse) network of fibres and cells permeating the isodendritic core of the brainstem and spinal grey matter and including the ascending and descending propriospinal fibre systems (Nauta and Karten, 1970). Like the long parvosynaptic (lemniscal) systems, this diffuse network also appears to have opiate and non-opiate links, but its organization is still too poorly understood to permit identification of two distinct categories.

The primary evidence for diffuse inhibitory controls is the well known fact that the excitatory receptive fields of many second order sensory neurones in the dorsal horn, particularly those with nociceptive input, can have a large inhibitory surround. Under some conditions, in fact, the inhibitory area may encompass essentially the whole body surface of the animal. Significantly, this diffuse inhibitory network is partly controlled by descending brainstem fibres, because severing the spinal cord can eliminate some of the inhibition in cells encountered at levels below the cut (Le Bars *et al.*, 1979).

Another example of widespread non-segmental inhibition, in this case involving primarily ascending fibres, is the suppression of the trigeminal jaw-opening reflex by electrical stimulation at distant points on the body surface (Tal *et al.*, 1981). A single electrical pulse delivered to the hindpaw, for example, increases the threshold for eliciting a jaw-opening reflex from tooth-pulp stimulation by as much as 500 ms. This effect is not blocked by naloxone. If one uses a prolonged train of electrical stimuli instead of single pulses then inhibition of the jaw-opening reflex can last for several minutes, and now becomes at least partially naloxone reversible. Some investigators have proposed that this so-called 'electro-acupuncture' is a useful model of traditional Chinese acupuncture (e.g. Toda and Ichioka, 1978).

SELECTIVITY OF DESCENDING CONTROL

It is generally agreed that the anti-nociceptive effects of electrical and pharmacological stimulation of periaqueductal grey are highly selective. Behavioural threshold to noxious thermal and mechanical stimuli increases without significant stupor or general sluggishness. Correspondingly (according to most reports), the response of wide dynamic range neurones in the dorsal horn to noxious stimuli is inhibited far more than their response to light touch; however, the selectivity is not absolute. Careful examination almost always shows up some depression of low threshold responses and according to some reports selectivity is at best modest (Duggan, 1982).

Three features of spinal cord functional organization make it almost inevitable that descending inhibition should act selectively on high threshold input. Firstly, the region of termination of nociceptive afferents in the most superficial layers of the dorsal horn, is also the area most densely populated with terminal of descending serotonergic fibres from the nucleus raphé magnus, and of descending adrenergic and peptidergic axons. This region is also rich in opiate receptors and local peptidergic interneurones.

Secondly, even if descending fibres did not terminate in special anatomical relationship with nociceptor endings, some degree of antinociceptive specificity would be expected. Synaptic inputs on to dorsal horn neurones are not all of equal strength. Low threshold input, especially near the centre of a cell's cutaneous receptive field, often has an extraordinarily high 'safety-factor' (defined as current available for excitation relative to current required). Often a single impulse in a single afferent is sufficient to produce repetitive discharge in the postsynaptic cell (Brown *et al.*, 1973). The synaptic efficacy of individual nociceptors is much lower. Furthermore, because of the rapid conduction velocity of low threshold afferents, natural touch stimuli produce a substantially coordinated input volley. Temporal convergence from slow conducting, high threshold afferents is much weaker. Thus, high threshold input is the more vulnerable to generalized pre- or postsynaptic inhibition especially if cells with particularly brisk low threshold responses are sampled.

The third reason that generalized descending inhibition would tend to be selectively anti-nociceptive concerns the excitatory receptive field structure of wide dynamic range neurones in lamina 5. Most such cells have convergent input at the centre of the receptive field and a purely high threshold input at the periphery (Wall, 1967). Furthermore, the peripheral input is relatively weak and when patient observations are made for example, one frequently finds spontaneous undulations of the borders of the receptive fields (Devor and Wall, 1981; and Figure 1.1). In some substantia gelatinosa neurones such 'amoeboid' variations are very pronounced (Dubuisson *et al.*, 1979). Furthermore, if one explores beyond the conventional field borders, there is often a substantial subliminal fringe of essentially unexpressed excitatory synaptic input. Many dorsal horn cells, for example, can be driven by electrical stimulation of afferents in nerves or dorsal roots that serve skin far distant from the borders of the receptive field. There is considerable evidence that under special experimental conditions the relatively ineffective inputs near and beyond the border can be strengthened, thus radically changing the spatial properties of the receptive field (Devor and Wall, 1981). In fact, it is possible that the intact central nervous system uses descending inhibitory controls to modulate field size and location.

Such control has consequences for stimulus quality and intensity coding and not merely for the coding of spatial properties of cutaneous stimuli. If all wide dynamic range receptive fields were expanded, then their overlap would ensure that stimulation at any given point would activate a large number of cells and dispatch a large impulse barrage supraspinally. If the fields were

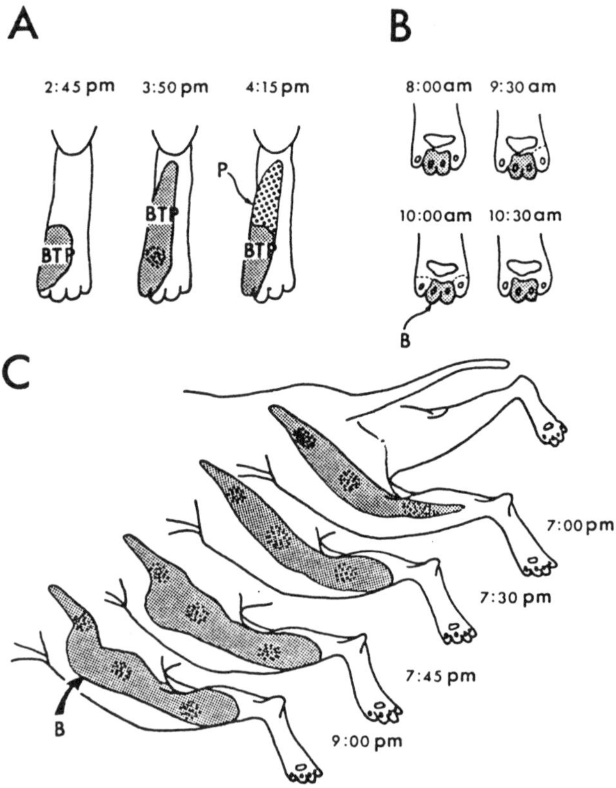

Figure 1.1 Spontaneous fluctutations in the receptive fields of three lamina 5 cells in intact cats. The time of each observation is indicated. (A) This cell initially responded to brushing of hairs, touch, and pressure (BTP) within the area indicated. Over the next hour its receptive field expanded proximally. In addition, a small zone appeared in which small movements of individual hairs strongly excited the cell (stippling). Subsequently this sensitive hair area disappeared, and the proximal half of the receptive field lost its sensitivity to brush and touch, remaining sensitive only to firm pressure (P), (B) This cell, responsive to hair brushing (B) on toes 2 and 3 acquired and then lost again response to hair movements on toes 1 and 4. At best, however, responses in these new areas were weak and habituated with repetition. (C) Receptive field borders of this brush-sensitive (B) cell undulated continuously. The three zones of sensitive hair response (stippling) were always present (reprinted from Devor and Wall (1981) with permission of the publishers).

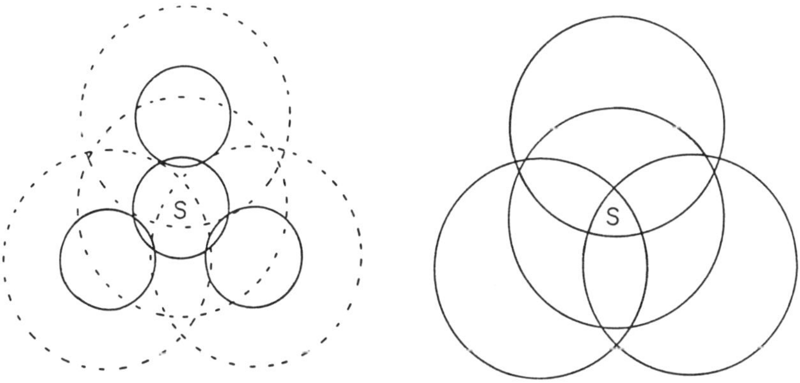

FIGURE 1.2 Spatial constriction of receptive field areas (circles) of dorsal horn neurones reduces field overlap. As a consequence, stimulation (S) at any given cutaneous site will activate fewer spinal projection neurones and the ascending sensory impulse barrage will be reduced correspondingly.

constricted, fewer cells would be excited and the ascending barrage would be correspondingly small (Figure 1.2).

EXPERIMENTAL ACCESS TO ENDOGENOUS PAIN CONTROL MECHANISMS

The selection pressures that led to the evolution of central pain control mechanisms presumably derive from the organism's need to perform even when faced with violence or the threat of violence. It should therefore be possible to activate these mechanisms experimentally by mimicking violence or the threat of violence. This approach, of course, is embodied in the literature on stress-induced analgesia (see reviews in the chapters that follow). An important distinction must be made, however, between actual violence and threat. There are several mechanisms whereby actual noxious stimuli could reduce pain responses by relatively simple short-loop negative feedback circuits. In contrast, responses to threat, which may be signalled either by actual injury or by subtler stimuli, are far more complicated. This is primarily because they involve an analysis of the *significance* of stimuli and the induction of anticipatory readiness states. Engagement of endogenous pain control mechanisms is only one component of such states.

Another means of experimental access to endogenous anti-nociceptive mechanisms is to activate them directly by electrophysiological or chemical means. Though the possibility of evoking organized behavioural or perceptual responses in an organ as complex as the brain may seem intuitively improbable the demonstration of stimulation bound feeding, drinking, copulatory behaviour, etc. illustrates the fruitfulness of this approach.

Finally, there appear to exist special psychological (including interoceptive) mechanisms that engage endogenous pain control systems, presumably by inducing central states similar to those induced in times of distress. Curiously, in man at least, relaxation and other correlates of the relief of distress also tend to be associated with analgesia. The survival value of such effects is not immediately obvious (but see Wall, 1979).

Noxious stimuli

With respect to actual tissue damage, at least two neural circuits have been identified that limit pain responses by negative feedback. The first circuit involves primary afferent input arriving in the spinal cord along low threshold (touch) fibres which inhibits ('gates') the responsiveness of second order transmission neurones to simultaneous high threshold input. Interneurones in the substantia gelatinosa are believed to be involved in this process (Melzack and Wall, 1965; Wall, 1978). Since most injuries activate both high and low threshold afferents, 'gate control' automatically limits the central response to noxious events.

The second proposed negative feedback route derives from the known excitation of cells in the nucleus raphé magnus by noxious stimulation over large areas of the body. Such excitation, of course, would potentiate the descending serotonergic pathway from the nucleus raphé magnus that inhibits high threshold afferent input at the level of the substantia gelatinosa (Basbaum and Fields, 1978). This bulbar negative feedback loop is almost certainly not exclusive to the nucleus raphé magnus pathway. In fact, very large receptive fields are a prominent characteristic of cells throughout the isodendritic core of the brainstem and spinal cord. Thus, many if not all descending and segmental inhibitory pathways are presumably influenced by negative feedback. Furthermore, since these same cells frequently receive polysensory (auditory, vestibular, visual, etc.) input and not purely somatosensory input, the activation of brainstem inhibitory mechanisms could well play a role in the analgesic effects of polysensory 'distracting' stimuli.

In addition to direct negative feedback mechanisms there is strong evidence that noxious stimuli can induce the local and/or systemic release of endogenous opiates. It is not clear, however, that this process is triggered *directly* by noxious stimuli rather than after the significance of these stimuli is evaluated at higher cerebral levels (see below). Indeed, recent findings pose challenging questions concerning the means by which stressful stimuli produce anti-nociceptive effects. Seemingly insignificant details of the stressful event have proved to have an important influence on the degree of analgesia, its spatial properties and its sensitivity to blockade or reversal by naloxone (e.g. Watkins and Mayer, 1982). A shock to the forepaws, for example, produces a very different analgesia than a shock to the hindpaws, and shocks that are inescapable have different effects than the same shocks delivered in an environment where escape is possible. Such observations are inconsistent with global release of opioids by noxious stimuli. In fact, there has been a tendency to propose separate endogenous pain control networks for each behavioural paradigm with the consequence that the number of such networks is increasing rapidly. Perhaps too much emphasis has been placed on the painful event itself, and not enough on its information content. What does a particular stressful stimulus portend? In the wild, would an injury (shock?) to the forepaw expose a rodent to the same type of dangers as an injury to the hindpaw?

Threats of violence

The sensory analysis of complex stimulus configurations, the evaluation of their behavioural significance, and the consequent activation of appropriate motor and autonomic responses requires data on higher cerebral functions about which modern neurophysiology still has precious little knowledge. It is these neural processes that presumably have the most powerful access to endogenous pain control circuitry. In the simplest case a noxious event might directly initiate defensive responses. In phylogenetically advanced species including man, however, stimuli capable of eliciting an emergency state can be extremely subtle, situation-dependent, and subject to conditioning and experience. Animals are superbly adapted to survival within a particular ecological niche, and their nervous systems are fine-tuned to evaluate situations portending violence in the environment in which they evolved. This must be kept in mind in any effort to find more effective non-pharmacological inducers of endogenous analgesia. To a desert snake, the sight of a mongoose is surely a much more relevant stressor than a 55 °C hot-plate. Correspondingly, electrical shocks in laboratory cages, convenient as they are to administer, may be poor substitutes for optimal stimuli for rodents. In this respect, recent experiments on stress associated with social conflicts in rats and mice (e.g. Kromer and Dum, 1980; Miczek *et al.*, 1982) are probably a step in the right direction.

Some years ago Komisaruk and Larsson (1971) showed a profound suppression of responses to noxious stimuli in female rats subjected to mechanical pressure on the uterine cervix. Apparently this suppression involves selective sensory gating and not merely simple flexor reflex inhibition. Endogenous opioids, however, have been clearly implicated in mating performance, where they might play a role both in anti-nociception and reward. Without doubt, the relation of sex to pain and stress merits further investigation. Indeed, just as pleasure and pain are in many ways two ends of a continuum, opiate-or 'state-'induced euphoria and analgesia may be expressions of a single mechanism. Finally, concern has frequently been expressed that standard laboratory rats have lost some of the fine tuning of their free-living cousins due to artificial (human) selection against the expression of emergency responses. Investigators of stress-induced phenomena might give more attention to hamsters, gerbils, voles, or other convenient species more recently introduced into the laboratory. The ethological literature on predator-prey interactions deals extensively with natural threats and has not been sufficiently considered (to the best of my knowledge) in relation to pain.

Ethical considerations

Inevitably, experimentation that involves doing or even threatening to do violence to laboratory animals raises important ethical questions and demands special justification. While even the most ardent animal defenders have not yet suggested that we protect forest rodents against hawks and owls, there is an obvious problem in our doing to rats in the laboratory what hawks do to rats in nature. We must remain always sensitive to this, and devise our experiments accordingly. The Committee for Research and Ethical Issues of the IASP (see *Pain,* **9** (1980), 141–4) has stressed that one should always keep in mind a humane balance between the amount of pain and suffering (and perhaps even anxiety) potentially inflicted on animals, and the value of the information likely to be gained toward the understanding and alleviation of pain and suffering in humans.

Electrical and chemical stimulation

As mentioned above, a search for brain loci at which focal electrical (or chemical) stimulation would have powerful anti-nociceptive effects led to the identification of the periaqueductal grey and associated nuclei as nodal points in descending pain control (Mayer and Liebeskind, 1974). It is noteworthy that several limbic forebrain structures, such as the lateral hypothalamus and septum, that have long been associated with reward, motivation, and affect, are intimately connected to the ventral periaqueductal grey by massive ascending and descending pathways.

A related way of gaining access to endogenous pain control mechanisms is to use drugs that have synaptic actions at critical points in the central pain mechanism. At present we know so little about the details of the central pain circuits that it is nearly impossible to design such drugs *a priori*. Fortunately, several classes of pharmacological agents long known for their analgesic actions are available for use as experimental probes. Without doubt, the most important such probes so far have been morphine and its derivatives. It was not long after specific receptor molecules were recognized as important for the mechanism of most drug actions, that specific morphine receptors were identified in neural tissue. The discoveries of endogenous ligands for opiate receptors (enkephalins, endorphins, and dynorphin), and the anatomical localization of opiate receptors and ligands in the brain and in the periphery came in rapid succession thereafter. It now appears likely that opioids play a role in a spectrum of different functional systems with actions locally in the CNS as classical neurotransmitters or neuromodulators, and also with actions as circulating neuro-hormones released by the pituitary and adrenal glands.

The existence of selective opiate antagonists (e.g. naloxone) has been a tremendous boon to research on the functional role of endogenous opiates. Any effect at least partially blocked by naloxone or its derivatives strongly suggests the involvement of endogenous opiate mechanisms. Such an assignation, however, is not as informative as it might appear. As discussed above, it is already well established that opiate receptors are widely distributed in the brain, and that opiate related synapses occur both close to the first central afferent synapse of nociceptors in the dorsal horn, and at the crucial interface between limbic forebrain and mid-brain structures. This being the case, all pain modulation phenomena are likely to be potentially influenced by opiates and/or their antagonists. The failure of an environmentally induced analgesia to be blocked or reversed by systemic naloxone means that endogenous opioid-dependent synapses are not obligatory components of the underlying neural circuit. It does not necessarily mean that they are not involved.

Interoceptive mechanisms

It is frankly surprising that higher cerebral levels have as little access to the central pain assembly as they do. Essentially automatic centrally programmed motor functions such as walking, chewing, breathing, and eye movements can be brought under voluntary control with great efficiency. By contrast, it seems to require effort and/or aptitude to overcome the reflex and perceptual manifestations of pain. However, higher cerebral access to the pain assembly obviously exists. This is clearly demonstrated by the well known analgesic potency of placebos and of hypnotic suggestion, and by the occasional dramatic success of faith healers, gurus and perhaps also of acupuncturists. The fact that these effects are highly unpredictable could simply indicate the subtle nature of the processes that intervene between the stimuli applied and the engagement of lower level anti-nociceptive circuitry. Once engaged, however, such psychologically induced analgesias may be subject to the same influences as simpler forms of analgesia. It has been claimed, for example, that the analgesic effects of acupuncture and placebo are at least partially blocked by naloxone (Mayer *et al.*, 1977; Levine *et al.*, 1978). It would not be too surprising if it turned out that some of the comforting effects of mother-love, for example, are likewise affected.

CONCLUSIONS

As part of the evolutionary process, mechanisms for modulating pain sensation and behavioural responses to pain have been built into the CNS. By consideration of the survival contingencies that favour the inhibition of pain, it is possible to predict what sorts of behavioural 'states' might be accompanied by analgesia: e.g. extreme fear, stress, aggressiveness, predation, sexual arousal, and defence. It is unlikely that environmental stimuli induce analgesia by simple and direct pathways. Rather, they convey information which is important for the survival of the organism. Analgesia should be considered as one of a constellation of anticipatory responses associated with complex behavioural 'states of readiness'.

REFERENCES

Basbaum, A. I., Marley, N. J. E., O'Keefe, J., and Clanton, C. H. (1977). Reversal of morphine and stimulus produced analgesia by subtotal spinal lesions. *Pain,* **3**, 43–56.

Basbaum, A. I., and Fields, H. L. (1978). Endogenous pain control mechanisms: review and hypothesis. *Annals Neurol.,* **4**, 451–462.

Beecher, H. K. (1956). Relationships of significance of wound to pain experienced. *J. Amer. Med. Assn.,* **161**, 1609–1613.

Brand, P. W. (1973). Rehabilitation of the hand with motor and sensory impairment. *Orthopedic Clinics of North America,* **4**, 1135–1139.

Brown, P. R., Moraff, H., and Tapper, D. N. (1973). Functional organization of the cat's dorsal horn: spontaneous activity and central cell response to single impulses in single type I fibers. *J. Neurophysiol.,* **36**, 827–839.

Carstens, E., Klumpp, D., and Zimmerman, M. (1979). The opiate antagonist naloxone does not affect descending inhibition from midbrain of nociceptive spinal neuronal discharges in the cat. *Neurosci. Lett.,* **11**,. 323–327.

Carstens, E., Mackinnon, J. D., and Guinan, M. J. (1982). Inhibition of spinal dorsal horn neuronal responses to noxious skin heating by medial preoptic and septal stimulation in the rat. *J. Neurophysiol.,* **48**, 981–991.

Devor, M., and Wall, P. D. (1981). The effect of peripheral nerve injury on receptive fields of cells in the cat spinal cord. *J. Comp. Neurol.,* **199**, 277–291.

Devor, M., and Govrin-Lippmann, R. (1983). Axoplasmic transport block reduces ectopic impulse generation in injured peripheral nerves. *Pain* **16**, 73–85.

Duggan, A. W. (1982). Brain stress control of the responses of spinal neurones to painful skin stimuli. *Trends in Neurosci.*, Apr. 127–130.

Dubuisson, D., Fitzgerald, M., and Wall, P. D. (1979). Ameboid receptive fields of cells in laminae 1, 2 and 3. *Brain Res.,* **177**, 376–378.

Fetz, E. E. (1968). Pyramidal tract effects on interneurons in the cat lumbar dorsal horn. *J. Neurophysiol.,* **31**, 69–80.

Fields, H. L., and Basbaum, A. I. (1978). Brainstem control of spinal pain-transmission neurons. *Ann. Rev. Physiol.,* **40**, 217–248.

Gamse, R., Holzer, P., and Lembeck, F. (1979). Indirect evidence for presynaptic location of opiate receptors on chemosensitive primary sensory neurones. *N.S. Arch. Pharmac.,* **308**, 281–285.

Gebhart, G. F. (1982). Opiate and opioid peptide effects on brainstem neurons: relevance to nociception and antinociceptive mechanisms. *Pain,* **12**, 93–140.

Glazer, E. J., and Basbaum, A. I. (1981). Immunohistochemical localisation of leucine-enkephalin in the spinal cord of the cat: enkephalin containing marginal neurons and pain modulation. *J. Comp. Neurol.*, **196**, 377–390.

Hagbarth, K. -E., and Kerr, D. I. B. (1954). Central influences on spinal afferent conduction. *J. Neurophysiol.*, **17**, 295–307.

Hebb, D. O. (1949). *Organization of Behaviour*, Wiley, New York.

Herkenham, M., and Pert, C. B. (1982). Light microscopic localization of brain opiate receptors: a general autoradiographic method which preserves tissue quality. *J. Neurosci.*, **2**, 1129–1149.

Komisaruk, B. R., and Larsson, K. (1971). Suppression of a spinal and cranial nerve reflex by vaginal or rectal probing in rats. *Brain Res.*, **35**, 231–235.

Kromer, W., and Dum, J. E. (1980). Mouse-killing in rats induces a naloxone-blockable increase in nociceptive threshold. *Europ. J. Pharmacol.*, **63**, 195–198.

Kruuk, H. (1964). Predators and anti-predator behaviour of the black-headed gull (*Larus ridibundus L.*). *Behav.*, **11**, 1–129.

Le Bars, D., Dickenson, A. H., and Besson, J. M. (1979). Diffuse noxious inhibitory controls (DNIC). I. Effects on dorsal horn convergent neurons in the rat. *Pain*, **6**, 283–304.

Levine, J. D., Gordon, N. C., and Fields, H. L. (1978). The mechanism of placebo analgesia. *Lancet*, **2**, 654–657.

Levine, J. D., Lane, S. R., Newton, C. G., and Fields, H. L. (1982). A spinal opioid synapse mediates the interaction of spinal and brainstem sites in morphine analgesia. *Brain Res.*, **236**, 85–91.

Mayer, D. J., and Liebeskind, J. C. (1974). Pain reduction by focal electrical stimulation of the brain: an anatomical and behavioural analysis. *Brain Res.*, **68**, 73–93.

Mayer, D. J., Price, D. D., and Rafii, A. (1977). Antagonism of acupuncture analgesia in man by the narcotic antagonist naloxone. *Brain Res.*, **121**, 368–372.

Melzack, R., and Wall, P. D. (1965). Pain mechanisms a new theory. *Science*, **150**, 971–978.

Miczek, K. A., Thompson, M. L., and Shuster, L. (1982). Opioid-like analgesia in defeated mice. *Science*, **215**, 1520–1522.

Nauta, W. J. H. (1958). Hippocampal projections and related neural pathways to the mid-brain in the cat. *Brain*, **81**, 319–340.

Nauta, W. J. H., and Karten, H. J. (1970). A general profile of the vertebrate brain, with sidelights on the ancestry of cerebral cortex, in *The Neuroscience: Second Study Program* (ed. F. O. Schmitt) Rockefeller U. Press, New York.

Penfield, W., and Rasmussen, T. (1950). *The Cerebral Cortex of Man*. Macmillan, New York.

Pretel, S., Frauhoffer, M., MacKinnon, J. D., and Carstens, E. (1982). Inhibition of spinal nociceptive transmission by cerebral cortical stimulation. *Neurosci. Abstr.*, **8**, 767.

Ratner, S. C. (1967). Comparative aspects of hypnosis, in *Handbook of Clinical and Experimental Hypnosis* (ed. J. E. Gordon). Macmillan, New York, pp. 550–587.

Sargent, C. B., and Eberhardt, L. E. (1975). Death feigning by ducks in response to predation by red foxes. *Am. Midl. Nat.*, **94**, 108–119.

Semmes, J. (1973). Somesthetic effects of damage to the central nervous system, in *Handbook of Sensory Physiology, Vol. II, Somatosensory System* (ed. A. Iggo), Springer-Verlag, Berlin.

Sherrington, C. S. (1906). *The Integrative Action of the Nervous System*, Yale University Press, New Haven.

Sweet, W. H. (1981). Animal models of chronic pain: their possible validation from human experience with posterior rhizotomy and congenital analgesia. *Pain,* **10**, 275–295.

Tal, M., Sharav, Y., and Devor, M. (1981). Modulation of the jaw-opening reflex by peripheral electrical stimulation. *Expt. Neurol.,* **74**, 907–919.

Toda, K., and Ichioka, M. (1978). Electroacupuncture: relations between forelimb afferent impulses and suppression of jaw-opening reflex in the rat. *Expt. Neurol.,* **61**, 465–470.

Wall, P. D. (1967). The laminar organization of dorsal horn and effects of descending impulses. *J. Physiol.,* **188**, 403–423.

Wall, P. D. (1978). The gate control theory of pain mechanisms: a re-examination and re-statement. *Brain,* **101**, 1–18.

Wall, P. D. (1979). On the relation of injury to pain: the John J. Bonica lecture. *Pain,* **6**, 253–264.

Watkins, L. R., and Mayer, D. J. (1982). Organization of endogenous opiate and nonopiate pain control systems. *Science,* **216**, 1185–1192.

Wyon-Maillard, M. -C., Conseiller, C., and Besson, J. -M. (1972). Effects of orbital cortex stimulation on dorsal horn interneurons in the cat spinal cord. *Brain Res.,* **46**, 71–83.

Yeung, J. C., and Rudy, T. A. (1980). Multiplicative interaction between narcotic agonisms expressed at spinal and supraspinal sites of antinociceptive action as revealed by concurrent intrathecal and intracerebroventricular injection of morphine. *J. Pharmacol. Exp. Ther.,* **215**, 633–642.

Stress-induced Analgesia
Edited by M. D. Tricklebank and G. Curzon

CHAPTER 2

Types of stress which induce analgesia

R. J. Bodnar

The concept of supraspinal modulation of spinal nociceptive input, originally proposed by Melzack and Wall (1965), now has considerable support, based on the observations that analgesia may be elicited following central electrical stimulation (Reynolds, 1969; Mayer *et al.*, 1971) or intracerebral microinjections of morphine (Tsou and Jang, 1964; Jacquet and Lajtha, 1973). Since stimulation-produced analgesia and morphine analgesia have some similarities, common physiological substrates have been proposed. As reviewed in detail elsewhere (Mayer and Price, 1976; Messing and Lytle, 1977; Yaksh and Rudy, 1978; Gebhart, 1982), both stimulation produced analgesia and morphine analgesia can be elicited from the periaqueductal grey, dorsal raphe nucleus, nucleus raphé magnus, and nucleus reticularis gigantocellularis. Both forms of analgesia exhibit tolerance, cross-tolerance, and synergy. Moreover, both are interrupted by lesions of either the dorsolateral funiculus of the spinal cord or the periaqueductal grey. Both forms of analgesia elicited from the periaqueductal grey excite units in the nucleus raphé magnus and inhibit units in the substantia gelatinosa of the spinal cord. However, while naloxone is agreed to eliminate morphine analgesia, opiate antagonism attenuates stimulation produced analgesia according to some (Akil *et al.*, 1976a; Oliveras *et al.*, 1977), but not to other (Yaksh *et al.*, 1976; Pert and Walter, 1976) studies.

From these and other data, Fields and Basbaum (1978) proposed that the projections between the periaqueductal grey, nucleus raphé magnus, and substantia gelatinosa comprised components of an opioid pain-inhibitory system. Based upon further data (see reviews: Yaksh, 1981; Watkins and Mayer, 1982), noradrenergic efferents through the nucleus reticularis gigantocellularis and nucleus alatus have also been implicated in the mediation of spinal analgesic responses.

These developments, together with the discoveries of the opiate receptor (Pert and Snyder, 1973; Simon *et al.*, 1973; Terenius, 1973) and the endogenous opioid ligands (Hughes *et al.*, 1975; Cox *et al.*, 1976; Guillemin *et al.*, 1976), spurred the search for endogenous and exogenous stimuli that might activate intrinsic pain-inhibitory systems. One explanation for the evolution of such systems is that they offer significant advantages for the survival of the organism in the processes of natural selection. There are many conceivable instances in which normal reactions to painful stimuli, e.g. withdrawal, rest and other recuperative behaviours could be seriously disadvantageous during predation, defence, confrontations for dominance, or acute adaptation to severe environmental demands. As noted by Cannon (1939), the responses to noxious or threatening stimuli is one of the basic adaptive mechanisms of animals and humans. Emergency situations are met by a number of autonomic adjustments of varying durations, such as changes in heart rate, muscle vasodilatation, pupillary dilatation, glucose and fat mobilization, constriction of capillary beds in the skin, and altered respiration, as well as by a complex, but integrated neuroendocrine response, involving pituitary-adrenal-cortical and sympatho-medullary activation (Selye, 1952). If pain-inhibitory systems were activated by such stimuli, one would expect analgesia to occur following acute exposure to them. The term 'stress-induced analgesia' has been used to describe this phenomenon. However, it must be realized that stress is neither a necessary nor sufficient condition to elicit analgesia, and that the environmental circumstances in which stress is applied may have a crucial role in the development of the decrease in response to pain. In this chapter, the types of stressors that induce analgesia will be reviewed. Emphasis will be placed upon the parameters employed and some comment will be made on the possible mechanisms involved. The latter issue is discussed at length in other chapters.

INITIAL STUDIES

In 1976, three laboratories (Akil *et al.*, 1976b; Hayes *et al.*, 1976; Rosecrans and Chance, 1976) reported that acute exposure to a stressful event increased pain thresholds. Akil and co-workers (Akil *et al.*, 1976b; Madden *et al.*, 1977) reported that acute exposure to inescapable footshock increased tail-flick latencies and appeared to increase endogenous opioids in brain as stereospecific opiate binding was inhibited. Daily chronic exposure to inescapable footshock over 10 days resulted in a diminution of both effects. Rosecrans and Chance (1976; Chance *et al.*, 1977, 1978) used inescapable footshock as an unconditioned stimulus and observed an increase in tail-flick latencies upon repeated presentation. The analgesic effect was also accompanied by significant inhibition of stereospecific opiate binding as well as by an increase in labelled leu-enkephalin binding in rat brain. Hayes and co-workers (1976, 1978a,b) found that acute exposure to a range of stressors, including inescapable footshock, centrifugal rotation and hypertonic saline injections, increased tail-flick latencies in rats with each stressor having its own characteristic effect on the magnitude and duration of the analgesic response.

However, stress (defined as a stimulus that activates the adrenocortical system) did not necessarily increase pain thresholds since neither ether inhalation nor horizontal oscillation increased tail-flick latencies following acute exposure. Moreover, despite the apparent association of analgesia due to inescapable footshock with opioid changes cited previously, Hayes and co-workers showed that the former effect was not altered by either a 1 mg/kg dose of naloxone or by lesions placed in the dorsolateral funiculus. In contrast, it was eliminated by spinalectomy suggesting the presence of some supraspinal control. These points will be discussed in detail in subsequent sections.

Following these initial observations, other environmental manipulations which are regarded as stressors were shown to increase pain thresholds, i.e. cold-water swims (Bodnar *et al.*, 1978a), injections of 2-deoxy-D-glucose (Bodnar *et al.*, 1978b), food deprivation (Bodnar *et al.*, 1978c), immobilization (Amir and Amit, 1978), insulin injections (Bodnar *et al.*, 1979a), heat exposure (Kulkarni, 1980), and body pinch (Ornstein and Amir, 1981). In contrast, tail-pinch increases pain thresholds using some tests of nociception (Levine *et al.*, 1982), but produces hyperalgesia using others (Simone and Bodnar, 1982). Furthermore, inescapable holding and novelty produce transient hyperalgesia (Vidal and Jacob, 1982). In subsequent sections, the analgesias induced by inescapable footshock, cold water swims, 2-deoxy-D-glucose, food deprivation, immobilization, and body pinch will be reviewed in detail.

INESCAPABLE FOOTSHOCK

As summarized previously, inescapable footshock produces analgesia following acute but not repeated exposure (Madden *et al.*, 1977). The initial attempts to correlate the analgesic response with alterations in endogenous opioids yielded results indicating that shock parameters, pain test, and the nature of opioid manipulation are important variables. In addition to inhibition of stereospecific opiate binding and increases in labelled leu-enkephalin binding, leu-enkephalin immunoreactivity in rat hypothalamus was decreased (Rossier *et al.*, 1978) while labelled met-enkephalin levels were unaltered (Fratta *et al.*, 1977). However, using naloxone to assess opioid involvement, footshock-induced increases in tail-flick latencies were blocked by a 10, but not by a 1 mg/kg dose (Akil *et al.*, 1976b; Hayes *et al.*, 1978a). Also footshock induced decreases in writhing in the mouse after i.p. administration of formic acid or PGE_1 were blocked by a 1 mg/kg dose (Chesher and Chan, 1977), but autoanalgesia in the rat was unaffected by a 10 mg/kg dose of naloxone (Chance and Rosecrans, 1979a). While morphine tolerance eliminated the reduction of writhing by inescapable footshock (Chesher and Chan, 1977), it failed to affect autoanalgesia (Chance and Rosecrans, 1979a).

If inescapable footshock is used as an unconditioned stimulus, successive presentations result in further increases in pain thresholds (autoanalgesia) rather than a return to baseline levels (Hayes *et al.*, 1978b; Chance *et al.*, 1978). Moreover, initial exposure to inescapable footshock also produced escape deficits 24–48 h thereafter (see review: Maier and Seligman, 1976; Weiss *et al.*, 1976; Anisman, 1977), Maier and colleagues (Jackson *et al.*, 1979; Maier *et al.*, 1979; Moye *et al.*, 1981) and brief re-exposure to inescapable footshock 24 h after initial exposure also produced an analgesic response. However, if the initial shocks were escapable, the subsequent analgesic effects were not observed (Maier *et al.*, 1982). Furthermore, rats observing other rats receiving inescapable footshock themselves show analgesia (Jensen and Smith, 1982).

Elegant experiments from several laboratories have demonstrated that parametric considerations are of crucial importance in assessing the mechanisms involved in the phenomenon. Lewis and co-workers (1980, 1981a) have shown that brief continuous inescapable footshock produced analgesia that was neither reversed by naloxone nor cross-tolerant with morphine but prolonged intermittent shock produced analgesia that was blocked by both procedures. Moreover, analgesia induced by the latter shock parameters are also blocked by dexamethasone pretreatment and by adrenal demedullation (Lewis *et al.*, 1980, 1982). Analgesias due to various schedules of inescapable footshock are blocked by hypophysectomy (Millan *et al.*, 1980) and by lesions placed in the arcuate nucleus of the hypothalamus (Przewlocki *et al.*, 1980), indicating an involvement of the hypothalamo–hypophysial portal system as well as its adrenocortical and sympatho-medullary components.

Somewhat similarly to the findings of Lewis *et al.*, Maier and co-workers found that increasing the number of 5 s shocks could differentially activate opioid and non-opioid dependent analgesias. Thus, exposure to 20 shocks produced analgesia that was not reversed by naltrexone but analgesia induced by 80 shocks was blocked (Grau *et al.*, 1981). Not only was the effect of prolonged exposure to inescapable footshock itself sensitive to opioid manipulations but also the analgesic response induced by brief re-exposure to footshock 24 h after prolonged inescapable footshock was reversible by naloxone and other opiate antagonists (Jackson *et al.*, 1979; Maier *et al.*, 1980), cross-tolerant with morphine (Drugan *et al.*, 1981) and attenuated in animals with alterations in the pituitary–adrenal axis (MacLennan *et al.*, 1982).

A third critical parameter in differentiating opioid and non-opioid involvement in shock-induced analgesia is the area of the body to which shock is applied. Watkins and Mayer (1982) found that shock delivered to the forepaws, but not to the hindpaws produced analgesia that was reversed by low doses of naloxone given either systemically or centrally and eliminated by lesions placed in the dorsolateral funiculus of the spinal cord or the nucleus raphé alatus (Watkins *et al.*, 1981). In contrast to the opioid-sensitive analgesia due to prolonged inescapable footshock, that induced by a brief series of shocks of relatively low intensity to the forepaws was unaffected in hypophysectomized rats (Watkins and Mayer, 1982). In like manner, autoanalgesia is also unaffected by these manipulations (Chance *et al.*, 1979; Watkins and Mayer, 1982). Further mechanisms of analgesia induced by inescapable footshock will be discussed in this volume in the chapters by Lewis and by Hutson *et al.*

COLD-WATER SWIMS

Following the initial studies with inescapable footshock, Kelly, Glusman and myself applied stress by subjecting rats to cold water swims and found a prolonged analgesic effect on the flinch-jump, tail-flick and operant liminal escape tests following acute exposure (Bodnar *et al.*, 1978a). Adaptation of the analgesic, but not of the hypothermic responses occurred following chronic exposure (Bodnar *et al.*, 1978d). Cold water swims in a 2°C bath for 3.5 min induced analgesia which was not cross-tolerant with morphine (Bodnar *et al.*, 1978e) nor eliminated by high doses of naloxone (Bodnar *et al.*, 1978f) suggesting that these conditions may activate a non-opioid pain-inhibitory system. In addition, although cold water swims are associated with changes of endogenous opioid peptide content (Pert and Bowie, 1979), the putative anti-enkephalinase, D-phenylalanine reduces its analgesic effects (Bodnar *et al.*, 1980a). Furthermore, the high affinity opiate antagonist naloxazone (Pasternak *et al.*, 1980) potentiates the analgesic effect of cold water swims while reducing morphine analgesia (Kirchgessner *et al.*, 1982). The latter studies suggest that opioid and non-opioid pain-inhibitory systems may act to inhibit one another under certain circumstances. Given the intrinsic importance of pain-inhibition, a collateral inhibitory system is intriguing since it implies the possibility that all analgesic mechanisms are not activated in response to a given stressor, but perhaps only those that are congruent with other complex responses that are simultaneously or subsequently elicited.

The above findings cannot necessarily be extrapolated to other conditions. For example, Christie and co-workers (1981, 1982a,b) found that after a 3 min swim in a 32°C bath, mice displayed analgesia in the writhing test that was cross-tolerant with morphine and correlated with labelled leu-enkephalin binding. We (Bodnar and Sikorszky, 1982) have found that naloxone can eliminate the analgesic response to a swim at 15°C. However, the analgesic effect of a 3.5 min swim at 2°C is decreased by naloxone only in animals that display a particularly large analgesic response. This suggests that larger analgesic responses may be mediated by both opioid and non-opioid mechanisms. The physiological basis of this individual variability in the magnitude of the analgesic response is unknown and obviously a matter for further study.

The non-opioid analgesic response following cold water swims is distinguishable from morphine analgesia in many ways. While hypophysectomy reduces the former effect, it potentiates the latter (Holaday *et al.*,, 1978; Bodnar *et al.*, 1979b). Moreover, Brattleboro rats (which have diabetes insipidus and vasopressin deficiency) display normal morphine analgesia but are without any analgesic response to cold water swims (Bodnar *et al.*, 1980b). Interestingly, vasopressin induces analgesia which is not antagonized by naloxone (Berntson and Berson, 1980; Kordower *et al.* 1982). In contrast, lesions of the serotonergic midbrain raphé nuclei or injection of the serotonin synthesis inhibitor parachlorophenylalanine prevents the analgesic effect of morphine, but not that of cold water swims (Tenen, 1968; Samanin *et al.*, 1970, 1973; Dostrovsky and Deakin, 1977; Brutus *et al.*, 1979; Bodnar *et al.*, 1981a). On the other hand, both types of analgesia are potentiated in adrenalectomized and neuroleptic-treated rats (Holaday *et al.*, 1979; Glusman *et al.*, 1980; Bodnar and Nicotera, 1982; Marek *et al.*, 1982) and are decreased in rats treated with apomorphine, tail-pinch, or neonatal monosodium glutamate (Bodnar *et al.*, 1980c,d; Simone and Bodnar, 1982). The latter manipulation destroys the cells of the hypothalamic arcuate nucleus and median eminence (see Olney, 1969) and may permanently impair responses to cold water swims as similarly treated rats also exhibit an impaired hypothermic response (Badillo-Martinez *et al.*, 1982). Therefore, although morphine and cold water swims appear to activate opioid and non-opioid pain-inhibitory mechanisms respectively, components of both systems appear to overlap.

2-DEOXY-D-GLUCOSE

This glucose analogue (Wick *et al.*, 1957; Himsworth, 1970) interferes with glucose metabolism causing hyperglycaemia and hyperphagia (Smith and Root, 1969; Smith and Epstein, 1969). It also produces analgesia following both systemic and central administration (Bodnar *et al.*, 1978b, 1981b). In common with the analgesic effect of cold water swims the stressful consequences of the treatment appear to be responsible for the analgesic response since this response and not the hyperphagia adapts on repeated 2-deoxyglucose injections (Bodnar *et al.*, 1978g). The analgesic response interacts with other stressors displaying cross-tolerance with the response to cold water swims and synergy with the response to food deprivation (Bodnar *et al.*, 1978b; Spiaggia *et al.*, 1979). However, unlike the analgesic response to cold water swims the response to 2-deoxyglucose exhibits both cross-tolerance and synergy with morphine analgesia (Spiaggia *et al.*, 1979; Bodnar *et al.*, 1979c). Both morphine and 2-deoxyglucose analgesias are decreased following lesions of the periaqueductal grey (Brutus *et al.*, 1979) and are potentiated in neuroleptic-treated or hypophysectomized rats (Bodnar *et al.*, 1979a; Bodnar and Nicotera, 1982), but neither naloxone nor parachlorophenylalanine altered 2-deoxyglucose analgesia (Bodnar *et al.*, 1979c, 1981a) and monosodium glutamate pretreatment potentiated it (Badillo-Martinez *et al.*, 1982). The latter manipulation also impaired the hyperphagic response to 2-deoxyglucose. The hyperphagic and analgesic responses to 2-deoxyglucose are further differentiated by their susceptibility to naloxone which decreases the former (Lowy *et al.*, 1980), but not the latter response (Bodnar *et al.*, 1979c). Furthermore, acute exposure to inescapable footshock eliminates the hyperphagic (Ritter *et al.*, 1978) but potentiates the analgesic effect of 2-deoxyglucose (unpublished data). Yet while repeated exposure to inescapable footshock does not alter the hyperphagic response to 2-deoxyglucose (Ritter *et al.*, 1978), the analgesia is eliminated by repeated pre-exposure to another stressor, cold water swims (Spiaggia *et al.*, 1979). Finally, if food is withheld for 6 h after giving 2-deoxyglucose to allow blood glucose levels to stabilize, rats still exhibit a hyperphagic (Bellin and Ritter, 1981), but not an analgesic response (unpublished data). Thus, the two main consequences of 2-deoxyglucose administration, analgesia and hyperphagia appear to be expressed through different physiological substrates.

FOOD DEPRIVATION

In initial studies using limited access to food, its deprivation had equivocal effects on pain thresholds (Dinsmoor, 1958; Franchina, 1966; Misanin and Campbell, 1969). However, to maximize steroid stress hormone alterations (Krieger, 1974), food deprivation should be abrupt. Therefore, when we (Bodnar *et al.*, 1978c) abruptly deprived rats of food over a 72 h period, flinch-jump thresholds increased after 12 h of deprivation if food was removed at the beginning of the dark cycle and after 12, 24, and 36 h of deprivation if food was removed at the beginning of the light cycle. Similar effects were obtained using the tail-flick test and the analgesia was shown to be antagonized by naloxone (McGivern *et al.*, 1979). The opioid component of food deprivation analgesia was present throughout a 24 h period despite changes in basal pain responsiveness (McGivern *et al.*, 1980). Analgesias due to food deprivation and 2-deoxyglucose exhibit synergy if tested in circumstances where 2-deoxyglucose is itself analgesic (Bodnar *et al.*, 1978b). Finally, though monosodium glutamate impairs other kinds of analgesia, it does not affect food deprivation analgesia (Bodnar *et al.*, 1980d).

IMMOBILIZATION CATALEPSY AND BODY PINCH

Amir and Amit (1978) demonstrated that restraint for up to 6 h produced increases in both tail-flick and hot-plate latencies which were blocked by moderate doses (4 mg/kg) of naloxone or hypophysectomy (Amir and Amit,

1979). Thus the analgesic effect of immobilization has similarities with those of prolonged inescapable footshock or cold water swims. The analgesia induced by immobilization cannot be attributed to deficits in motor performance since this is not detectably impaired (Blair *et al.*, 1982). Catalepsy is also associated with analgesia. Thus, animals are both cataleptic and analgesic following an electroconvulsive shock, and both states are reduced by naloxone analgesia (Belenky and Holaday, 1979; Holaday and Belenky, 1980; Lewis *et al.*, 1981b). Furthermore, in the resident-intruder model of aggression, the intruder displays catalepsy and analgesia when attacked, effects which are reversible by naloxone (Miczek *et al.*, 1982) while repeated body pinches to mice, particularly around the scruff of the neck, produce gradual analgesic and cataleptic effects which are blocked by opiate antagonists (Ornstein and Amir, 1981).

SUMMARY

The discovery that certain environmental events can activate endogenous pain-inhibitory systems has led to many new insights into analgesic processes. Though some of the analgesic responses following these stimuli are similar to those induced by opiates, it is now clear that both opioid and non-opioid pain-inhibitory systems exist and that different environmental stressors produce different effects because they are activating different analgesia systems. Furthermore, a single stressor may activate (or otherwise alter) more than one analgesic system. Finally, individual differences in analgesic responses (like other coping responses to stress) are important in assessing physiological mechanisms and may help to provide models for the activation of different analgesic systems. Future research might profitably use known types of stress-induced analgesia to elucidate further the underlying substrates that activate, modulate and express nociceptive processes.

ACKNOWLEDGEMENT

I thank Drs Dennis Kelly and Murray Glusman for their friendly collaboration in the work of our laboratory and also the undergraduate and graduate students who worked on these projects at the New York State Psychiatric Institute and Queens College, CUNY.

REFERENCES

Akil, H., Mayer, D. J., and Liebeskind, J. C. (1976a). Antagonism of stimulation-produced analgesia by naloxone, a narcotic antagonist. *Science,* **191**,. 961–963.

Akil, H., Madden, J., Patrick, R. L., and Barchas, J. D. (1976b). Stress-induced increase in endogenous opiate peptides: concurrent analgesia and its partial reversal by naloxone, in *Opiate and Endogenous Opiate Peptides* (ed. H. W. Kosterlitz), North-Holland, Amsterdam.

Amir, S., and Amit, Z. (1978). Endogenous opioid ligands may mediate stress-induced changes in the affective properties of pain related behavior in rats. *Life Sci.,* **23**, 1143–1152.

Amir, S., and Amit, Z. (1979). The pituitary gland mediates acute and chronic pain responsiveness in stressed and non-stressed rats. *Life Sci.,* **24**, 439–448.

Anisman, H. (1977). Time-dependent changes in activity, reactivity and responsivity during shock: effects of cholinergic and catecholaminergic manipulations. *Behav. Biol.,* **21**, 1–31.

Badillo-Martinez, D., Nicotera, N., Butler, P., Kirchgessner, A. L., Sperber, E., and Bodnar, R. J. (1982). Characterization of stress-related responses in the monosodium glutamate treated rat. *Soc. Neurosci. Abstr.,* **8**, 621.

Belenky, G. L., and Holaday, J. W. (1979). The opiate antagonist naloxone modifies the effects of electroconvulsive shock (ECS) on respiration, blood pressure and heart rate. *Brain Res.,* **177**, 414–417.

Bellin, S. I., and Ritter, S. (1981). Disparate effects of infused nutrients on delayed glucoprivic feeding and hypothalamic norepinephrine turnover. *J. Neurosci.,* **1**, 1347–1353.

Berntson, G. G., and Berson, B. S. (1980). Antinociceptive effects of intraventricular or systemic administration of vasopressin in the rat. *Life Sci.,* **26**, 455–459.

Blair, R., Galina, Z. H., Holmes, L. J., and Amit, Z. (1982). Stress-induced analgesia: a performance deficit or a change in pain responsiveness. *Behav. Neur. Biol.,* **34**, 152–158.

Bodnar, R. J., Kelly, D. D., and Glusman, M. (1978a). Stress-induced analgesia: time course of pain reflex alterations following cold-water swims. *Bulletin of the Psychonomic Society,* **11**, 333–336.

Bodnar, R. J., Kelly, D. D., Brutus, M., Mansour, A., and Glusman, M. (1978b). 2-Deoxy-D-glucose-induced decrements in operant and reflex pain thresholds. *Pharmac. Biochem. Behav.,* **9**, 543–549.

Bodnar, R. J., Kelly, D. D., Spiaggia, A., and Glusman, M. (1978c). Biphasic alterations of nociceptive thresholds induced by food deprivation. *Physiological Psychology,* **6**, 391–395.

Bodnar, R. J., Kelly, D. D., Spiaggia, A., and Glusman, M. (1978d). Stress-induced analgesia: adaptation following chronic cold-water swims. *Bulletin of the Psychonomic Society,* **11**, 337–340.

Bodnar, R. J., Kelly, D. D., Steiner, S. S., and Glusman, M. (1978e). Stress-produced analgesia and morphine-produced analgesia: lack of cross-tolerance. *Pharmac. Biochem., Behav.,* **8**, 661–666.

Bodnar, R. J., Kelly, D. D., Spiaggia, A., Ehrenberg, C., and Glusman, M. (1978f). Dose-dependent reductions by naloxone of analgesia induced by cold-water stress. *Pharmac. Biochem. Behav.,* **8**, 667–672.

Bodnar, R. J., Kelly, D. D., Brutus, M., and Glusman, M. (1978g). Chronic 2-deoxy-D-glucose treatment: adaptation of its analgesic, but not hyperphagic properties. *Pharmac. Biochem. Behav.,* **9**, 763–768.

Bodnar, R. J., Kelly, D. D., Mansour, A., and Glusman, M. (1979a). Differential effects of hypophysectomy upon analgesia induced by two glucoprivic stressors and morphine. *Pharmac. Biochem. Behav.,* **11**, 303–307.

Bodnar, R. J., Glusman, M., Brutus, M., Spiaggia, A., and Kelly, D. D. (1979b). Analgesia induced by cold-water stress: attenuation following hypophysectomy. *Physiol. Behav.,* **23**, 53–62.

Bodnar, R. J., Kelly, D. D., and Glusman, M. (1979c). 2-Deoxy-D-glucose analgesia:

influences of opiate and non-opiate factors. *Pharmac. Biochem. Behav.*, **11**, 297–301.

Bodnar, R. J., Lattner, M., and Wallace, M. M. (1980a). Antagonism of stress-induced analgesia by D-phenylalanine, an anti-enkephalinase. *Pharmac. Biochem. Behav.*, **13**, 829–833.

Bodnar, R. J., Zimmerman, E. A., Nilaver, G., Mansour, A., Thomas, L. W., Kelly, D. D., and Glusman, M. (1980b). Dissociation of cold-water swim and morphine analgesia in Brattleboro rats with diabetes insipidus. *Life Sci.*, **26**, 1581–1590.

Bodnar, R. J., Kelly, D. D., Brutus, M., Greenman, C. B., and Glusman, M. (1980c). Reversal of stress-induced analgesia by apomorphine, but not by amphetamine. *Pharmac. Biochem. Behav.*, **13**, 171–175.

Bodnar, R. J., Abrams, G. W., Zimmerman, E. A., Krieger, D. T., Nicholson, G., and Kizer, J. S. (1980d). Neonatal monosodium glutamate: effects upon analgesic responsivity and immunocytochemical ACTH/B-lipotropin. *Neuroendocrinology*, **30**, 280–284.

Bodnar, R. J., Kordower, J. H., Wallace, M. M., and Tamir, H. (1981a). Stress and morphine analgesia: alterations following *p*-chlorophenylalanine. *Pharmac. Biochem. Behav.*, **14**, 645–651.

Bodnar, R. J., Merrigan, K. P., and Wallace, M. M. (1981b). Analgesia following intraventricular administration of 2-deoxy-D-glucose. *Pharmac. Biochem. Behav.*, **14**, 579–581.

Bodnar, R. J., and Nicotera, N. (1982). Neuroleptic and analgesic interactions upon pain and activity measures. *Pharmac. Biochem. Behav.*, **16**, 411–416.

Bodnar, R. J., and Sikorszky, V. Naloxone and cold-water swim analgesia: parametric considerations and individual differences. *Learning and Motiv.*, in review.

Bolles, R. C., and Fanselow, M. S. (1980). A perceptual-defensive-recuperative model of fear and pain. *Behav. and Brain Sci.*, **3**, 291–323.

Brutus, M., Kelly, D. D., Glusman, M., and Bodnar, R. J. (1979). Periaqueductal gray lesions and non-narcotic anti-nociception. *Soc. Neurosci. Abstr.*, **5**, 606.

Cannon, W. B. (1939). *The Wisdom of the body*, Norton, New York.

Chance, W. T., Krynock, G. M., and Rosecrans, J. A. (1978). Antinociception following lesion-induced hyperemotionality and conditioned fear. *Pain*, **4**, 243–252.

Chance, W. T., and Rosecrans, J. A. (1979a). Lack of effect of naloxone on autoanalgesia. *Pharmac. Biochem. Behav.*, **11**, 643–646.

Chance, W. T., and Rosecrans, J. A. (1979b). Lack of cross-tolerance between morphine and autoanalgesia. *Pharmac. Biochem. Behav.*, **11**, 639–642.

Chance, W. T., White, A. C., Krynock, G. M., and Rosecrans, J. A. (1977). Autoanalgesia: behaviorally activated antinociception. *Europ. J. Pharmac.*, **44**, 283–284.

Chance, W. T., Krynock, G. M., and Rosecrans, J. A. (1979). Investigation of pituitary influences on autoanalgesia. *Psychoneuroendocrinol.*, **4**, 199–205.

Chesher, G. B., and Chan, B. (1977). Footshock induced analgesia in mice: its reversal by naloxone and cross tolerance with morphine. *Life Sci.*, **21**, 1569–1574.

Christie, M. J., Chesher, G. B., and Bird, K. D. (1981). The correlation between swim-stress induced antinociception and [^{3}H] leu-enkephalin binding to brain homogenates in mice. *Pharmac. Biochem. Behav.*, **15**, 853–857.

Christie, M. J., and Chesher, G. B. (1982a). Physical dependence on physiologically released endogenous opiates. *Life Sci.*, **30**, 1173–1177.

Christie, M. J., Trisdikoon, P., and Chesher, G. B. (1982b). Tolerance and cross tolerance with morphine resulting from physiological release of endogenous opiates. *Life Sci.*, **31**, 839–845.

Cox, B. M., Goldstein, A., and Li, C. H. (1976). Opioid activity of a peptide B-lipotropin (61–91) derived from B-lipotropin. *Proc. nat. Acad. Sci.* (Wash.), **73**, 1821–1823.

Dinsmoor, J. A. (1958). Pulse duration and food deprivation in escape-from-shock training. *Psycholog. Rep.,* **4**, 531–534.

Dostrovsky, J. O., and Deakin, J. F. W. (1977). Periaqueductal grey lesions reduce morphine analgesia in the rat. *Neuroscience Letters,* **4**, 99–103.

Drugan, R. C., Grau, J. W., Maier, S. F., Madden, J., and Barchas, J. D. (1981). Cross tolerance between morphine and the long-term analgesic reaction to inescapable shock. *Pharmac. Biochem. Behav.,* **14**, 677–682.

Fanselow, M. S. (1981). Naloxone and Pavlovian fear conditioning. *Learning and Motivation,* **12**, 398–419.

Fields, H., and Basbaum, A. (1978). Brainstem control of spinal pain transmission neurons. *Ann. Rev. Physiol.,* **40**, 217–248.

Franchina, J. J. (1966). Combined sources of motivation and escape responding. *Psychonomic Sci.,* **6**, 221–222.

Fratta, W., Yang, H. Y. T., Hong, J., and Costa, E. (1977). Stability of met-enkephalin content in brain structures of morphine-dependent or foot-shocked rats. *Nature,* **268**, 452–453.

Gebhart, G. F. (1982). Opiate and opioid peptide effects on brain stem neurons: relevance to nociception and antinociceptive mechanisms. *Pain,* **12**, 93–140.

Glusman, M., Bodnar, R. J., Mansour, A., and Kelly, D. D. (1980). Enhancement of stress-induced analgesia by adrenalectomy in the rat. *Soc. Neurosci. Abstr.,* **6**, 321.

Grau, J. W., Hyson, R. L., Maier, S. F., Madden, J., IV, and Barchas, J. D. (1981). Long-term stress-induced analgesia and activation of the opiate system. *Science,* **213**, 1409–1411.

Guillemin, R., Ling, N., and Burgus, R. (1976). Endorphins, hypothalamic neurohypophysial peptides with morphomemetic activity. Isolation and primary structure of alpha-endorphin, *C. R. Acad. Sci.* (Paris), **282**, 783–785.

Hayes, R. L., Bennett, G. J., Newlon, P., and Mayer, D. J. (1976). Analgesic effects of certain noxious and stressful manipulations in the rat. *Soc. Neurosci. Abstr.,* **2**, 1350.

Hayes, R. L., Price, D. D., Bennett, G. J., Wilcox, G. L., and Mayer, D. J. (1978a). Differential effects of spinal cord lesions on narcotic and non-narcotic suppression of nociceptive reflexes: further evidence for the physiologic multiplicity of pain modulation. *Brain Res.,* **155**, 91–101.

Hayes, R. L., Bennett, G. J., Newlon, P. G., and Mayer, D. J. (1978b). Behavioral and physiological studies of non-narcotic analgesia in the rat elicited by certain environmental stimuli. *Brain Res.,* **155**, 69–90.

Himsworth, R. L. (1970). Hypothalamic control of adrenaline secretion in reponse to insufficient glucose. *J. Physiol.* (Lond.), **198**, 451–465.

Holaday, J. W., Law, P. Y., Tseng, L. F., Loh, H. H., and Li, C. H. (1978). B-endorphin: pituitary and adrenal glands modulate its action. *Proc. Natl Acad. Sci.,* **74**, 4628–4632.

Holaday, J. W., Law, P. Y., Loh, H. H., and Li, C. H. (1979). Adrenal steroids indirectly modulate opiate sensitivity. *J. Pharmac. exp. Ther.,* **208**, 176–183.

Holaday, J. W., and Belenky, G. L. (1980). Opiate-like effects of electroconvulsive shock in rats: a differential effect of naloxone on nociceptive measures. *Life Sci.,* **27**, 1929–1938.

Hughes, J., Smith, T., Kosterlitz, H. W., Fothergill, L. A., Morgan, B. A., and Morris, H. R. (1975). Identification of two related penta-peptides from the brain with potent opiate agonist activity. *Nature* (Lond.), **258**, 577–579.

Jackson, R. L., Maier, S. F., Coon, D. J. (1979). Long-term analgesic effects of inescapable shock and learned helplessness. *Science,* **206**, 91–93.

Jacquet, Y. F., and Lajtha, A. (1973). Morphine action at central nervous system sites in the rat: analgesia or hyperalgesia depending on site and dose. *Science,* **182**, 490–492.

Jensen, T. S., and Smith, D. F. (1982). Dopaminergic effects on tail-flick response in spinal rats. *Eur. J. Pharmac.,* **79**, 129–133.

Kirchgessner, A. L., Bodnar, R. J., and Pasternak, G. W. (1982). Naloxazone and pain-inhibitory systems: evidence for a collateral inhibition model. *Pharmac. Biochem. Behav.,* **17**, 1175–1179.

Kordower, J. H., Sikorszky, V., and Bodnar, R. J. (1982). Central antinociceptive effects of lysine-vasopressin and an analogue. *Peptides,* **3**, 613–617.

Krieger, D. T. (1974). Food and water restriction shifts corticosterone, temperature, activity and brain amine periodicity. *Endocrinology,* **95**, 1195–1201.

Kulkarni, S. K. (1980). Heat and other physiological stress-induced analgesia: catecholamine mediated and naloxone reversible response. *Life Sci.,* **27**, 185–188.

Levine, A. S., Wilcox, G. L., Grace, M., and Morley, J. E. (1982). Tail pinch induced consummatory behaviors are associated with analgesia. *Physiol. Behav.,* **28**, 959–962.

Lewis, J. W., Cannon, J. T., and Liebeskind, J. C. (1980). Opioid and non-opioid mechanisms of stress analgesia. *Science,* **208**, 623–625.

Lewis, J. W., Sherman, J. E., and Liebeskind, J. C. (1981a). Opioid and non-opioid stress analgesia: assessment of tolerance and cross-tolerance with morphine. *J. Neurosci.,* **1**, 358–363.

Lewis, J. W., Cannon, J. T., Chudler, E. H., and Liebeskind, J. C. (1981b). Effects of naloxone and hypophysectomy on electro-convulsive shock-induced analgesia. *Brain Res.,* **208**, 230–233.

Lewis, J. W., Tordoff, M. G., Sherman, J. E., and Liebeskind, J. C. (1982). Adrenal medullary enkephalin-like peptides may mediate opioid stress analgesia. *Science,* **217**, 557–559.

Lowy, M. T., Maickel, R. P., and Yim, G. K. W. (1980). Naloxone reduction of stress-related feeding. *Life Sci.,* **26**, 2113–2118.

MacLennan, A. J., Drugan, R. C., Hyson, H. L., Maier, S. F., Madden, J., and Barchas, J. D. (1982). Corticosterone: a critical factor in an opioid form of stress-induced analgesia. *Science,* **215**, 1530–1532.

Madden, J., Akil, H., Patrick, R. L., and Barchas, J. D. (1977). Stress-induced parallel changes in central opioid levels and pain responsiveness in the rat. *Nature,* **265**, 358–360.

Maier, S. F., and Seligman, M. E. P. (1976). Learned helplessness: theory and evidence. *J. exp. Psych.* (Gen.),. **105**, 3–46.

Maier, S. F., Coon, D. J., McDaniel, M. A., Jackson, R. L., and Grau, J. (1979). The time course of learned helplessness, inactivity and nociceptive deficits in rats. *Learning and Motiv.,* **10**, 467–487.

Maier, S. F., Davies, S., Grau, J. W., Jackson, R. L., Morrison, D. H., Moye, T., Madden, J., and Barchas, J. D. (1980). Opiate antagonists and long-term analgesic reaction induced by inescapable foot shock. *J. comp. physiol. Psych.,* **94**, 1172–1183.

Maier, S. F., Drugan, R. C., and Grau, J. C. (1982). Controlability, coping behavior and stress-induced analgesia in the rat. *Pain,* **12**, 47–56.

Marek, P., Ponocka, I., and Hartmann, G. (1982). Enhancement of stress-induced analgesia in adrenalectomized mice: its reversal by dexamethasone. *Pharmac. Biochem. Behav.,* **16**, 403–405.

Mayer, D. J., and Price, D. D. (1976). Central nervous system mechanisms of analgesia. *Pain,* **2**, 379–404.

Mayer, D. J., Wolfle, T. L., Akil, H., Carder, B., and Liebeskind, J. C. (1971). Analgesia from electrical stimulation in the brainstem of the rat. *Science,* **174**, 1351–1354.

McGivern, R., Berka, C., Berntson, G. G., Walker, J. M., and Sandman, C. A. (1979). Effect of naloxone on analgesia induced by food deprivation. *Life Sci.,* **25**, 885–888.

McGivern, R. F., and Berntson, G. G. (1980). Mediation of diurnal fluctutations in pain sensitivity in the rat by food intake patterns: reversal by naloxone. *Science,* **210**, 210–211.

Melzack, R., and Wall, P. D. (1965). Pain mechanisms: a new theory. *Science,* **150**, 971–979.

Messing, R. B., and Lytle, L. D. (1977). Serotonin-containing neurons: their possible role in pain and analgesia. *Pain,* **4**, 1–21.

Miczek, K. A., Thompson, M. L., and Shuster, L. (1982). Opioid-like analgesia in defeated mice. *Science,* **215**, 1518–1520.

Millan, M. J., Przewlocki, R., and Herz, A. (1980). A non B-endorphinergic adrenohypophyseal mechanism is essential for an analgetic response to stress. *Pain,* **8**, 343–353.

Misanin, J. R., and Campbell, B. A. (1969). Effects of hunger and thirst on sensitivity and reactivity to shock. *J. Comp. Physiol. Psychol.,* **69**, 207–213.

Moye, T. B., Coon, D. J., Grau, J. W., and Maier, S. F. (1981). Therapy and immunization of long-term analgesia in rats. *Learning and Motivation,* **12**, 133–148.

Oliveras, J. L., Hosobuchi, Y., Redjemi, F., Guilbaud, G., and Besson, J. M. (1977). Opiate antagonist, naloxone, strongly reduces analgesia induced by stimulation of a raphe nucleus (centralis inferior). *Brain Res.,* **120**, 221–229.

Olney, J. W. (1969). Brain lesions, obesity and other disturbances in mice treated with monosodium glutamate. *Science,* **164**, 719–721.

Ornstein, K., and Amir, S. (1981). Pinch-induced catalepsy in mice. *J. Comp. Physiol. Psychol.,* **95**, 827–835.

Pasternak, G. W., Childers, S. R., and Snyder, S. H. (1980). Opiate analgesia: evidence for mediation by a subpopulation of opiate receptors. *Science,* **208**, 514–516.

Pert, C., and Snyder, S. H. (1973). Opiate receptor: demonstration in nervous tissue., *Science,* **179**, 1011–1014.

Pert, A, and Walter, M. (1976). Comparison between naloxone reversal of morphine and electrical stimulation induced analgesia in the rat mesencephalon. *Life Sci.,* **19**, 1023–1032.

Pert, C. B., and Bowie, D. L. (1979). Behavioral manipulation of rats causes alterations in opiate receptor occupancy, in *Endorphins in Mental Health Research* (eds E. Usdin, W. E. Bunney, and N. S. Kline), pp. 93–104, Oxford, New York.

Przewlocki, R., Millan, M. J., and Herz, A. (1980). Is B-endorphin involved in analgesia generated by stress, in *Endogenous and Exogenous Opiate Agonists and Antagonists* (ed. E. L. Way), pp. 391–394, Pergamon, New York.

Reynolds, D. V. (1969). Surgery in the rat during electrical analgesia induced by focal brain stimulation. *Science,* **164**, 444–445.

Ritter, S., Pelzer, N. L., and Ritter, R. C. (1978). Absence of glucoprivic feeding after stress suggests impairment of noradrenergic neuron function. *Brain Res.,* **149**, 399–411.

Rosecrans, J. A., and Chance, W. T. (1976). Emotionality-induced antinociception. *Soc. Neurosci. Abstr.,* **2**, 919.

Rossier, J., Guilleman, R., and Bloom, F. (1978). Foot shock induced stress decreases Leu^5-enkephalin immunoreactivity in rat hypothalamus. *Eur. J. Pharmac.,* **48**, 465–466.

Samanin, R., Gulmulka, W., and Valzelli, L. (1970). Reduced effect of morphine in midbrain raphe lesioned rats. *Europ. J. Pharmacol.,* **10**, 339–343.

Samanin, R., Ghezzi, D., Mauron, C., and Valzelli, L. (1973). Effect of midbrain raphe lesion on the antinociceptive action of morphine and other analgesics in rats. *Psychopharm.,* **33**, 365–368.

Selye, H. (1952). *The Story of the Adaptation Syndrome*, Acta Inc., Montreal.

Simon, E. J., Hiller, J. M., and Edelman, I. (1973). Stereospecific binding of the potent narcotic ^{3}H-etorphine to rat brain homogenate. *Proc. Natl Acad. Sci. USA,* **70**, 1947–1949.

Simone, D. A., and Bodnar, R. J. (1982). Modulation of antinociceptive responses following tail pinch stress. *Life Sci.,* **30**, 719–729.

Smith, G. P., and Epstein, A. N. (1969). Increased feeding in response to decreased glucose utilization in the rat and monkey. *Am. J. Physiol.,* **217**, 1083–1087.

Smith, G. P., and Root, A. W. (1969). Effect of feeding on hormonal responses to 2-deoxy-D-glucose in conscious monkeys. *Endocrinology,* **85**, 963–966.

Spiaggia, A., Bodnar, R. J., Kelly, D. D., and Glusman, M. (1979). Opiate and non-opiate mechanisms of stress-induced analgesia: cross-tolerance between stressors. *Pharmac. Biochem. Behav.,* **10**, 761–765.

Tenen, S. S. (1968). Antagonism of the analgesic effect of morphine and other drugs by *p*-chlorophenylalanine, a serotonin depletor. *Psychopharm.,* **12**, 278–285.

Terenius, L. (1973). Stereospecific interaction betwen narcotic analgesics and a synaptic plasma membrane fraction of rat cerebral cortex. *Acta Pharmacol. Toxicol.,* **32**, 317–320.

Tsou, K., and Jang, C. S. (1964). Studies on the site of analgesic action of morphine by intracerebral microinjection. *Sci. sin.,* **13**, 1099–1109.

Vidal, C., and Jacob, J. J. C. (1982). Stress hyperalgesia in rats: an experimental animal model of anxiogenic hyperalgesia in human. *Life Sci.,* **31**, 1241–1244.

Watkins, L. R., and Mayer, D. J. (1982). The neural organization of endogenous opiate and non-opiate pain control systems. *Science,* **216**, 1185–1192.

Watkins, L. R., Young, E. G., Kinscheck, I. B., and Mayer, D. J. (1981). Effect of n. raphe alatus and periaqueductal gray lesions on footshock induced analgesia and classically conditioned analgesia. *Soc. Neurosci. Abstr.,* **7**, 533.

Weiss, J. M., Glazer, H. I., and Pohorecky, L. A. (1976). Coping behavior and neurochemical changes: an alternative explanation for the original 'learned helplessness' experiments, in *Animal Models in Human Psychobiology* (eds G. Serban and A. Kling), pp. 124–160, Plenum, New York.

Wick, A. N., Drury, D. R., Nakada, H. I., and Wolfe, J. B. (1957). Localization of the primary metabolic block produced by 2-deoxy-D-glucose. *J. biol. Chem.,* **224**, 963–969.

Yaksh, T. L. (1981). Spinal opiate analgesia: characteristics and principles of action. *Pain,* **11**, 293–346.

Yaksh, T. L., and Rudy, T. A. (1978). Narcotic analgesics: CNS sites and mechanisms of action as revealed by intracerebral injection techniques. *Pain*, **4**, 299–359.

Yaksh, T. L., Yeung, J. C., and Rudy, T. A. (1976). An inability to antagonize with naloxone the elevated nociceptive thresholds resulting from electrical stimulation of the mesencephalic central gray. *Life Sci.,* **18**, 1193–1198.

Stress-induced Analgesia
Edited by M. D. Tricklebank and G. Curzon

CHAPTER 3

Motor, motivational and anti-nociceptive consequences of stress: contribution of neurochemical changes

R. M. Zacharko and H. Anisman

When subjected to physical insults, animals tend to engage in behaviours that serve to minimize their impact. These adaptive responses often take the form of species-specific defensive behaviours, such as freezing, fleeing, or fighting (Bolles, 1970). The response shown at any particular time presumably reflects its position in an hierarchy of defensive behaviours. If the initial response does not eliminate the aversive stimulation then another kind of response will occur and so on until the most effective strategy within the repertoire is found.

Appropriate responses which are not part of this repertoire, can be learned through instrumental means though the ease with which this occurs is also species dependent. For example, some species (e.g., rats and mice) learn unidirectional more readily than bidirectional responses, whereas other species (e.g., gerbils) are equally able to learn either type of response (Ashe and McCain, 1972). Also, rats learn to jump on to a ledge against a wall of a test chamber more readily than they learn to jump on to one at the centre of the chamber (Grossen and Kelley, 1972), while arboreal and terrestrial mice respectively adopt jumping and running responses with greatest facility (see Bignami and Michalek, 1978; Wahlsten, 1980).

Also, some stimulus-response associations are acquired more readily than others (Shettleworth, 1972). Moreover, spatial and temporal relationships between the warning and aversive stimuli may affect the rapidity with which a defensive strategy is established (Testa, 1974). The essential points here are that many defensive styles are available to animals and that the coping strategy selected may be species specific. Thus, behaviours motivated by aversive stimulation, may be dictated by unconditioned responses inherent to the particular species or strain under investigation.

Neurochemical, hormonal, and immunological changes also occur in response to stress and are similarly thought to have adaptive significance (Sklar and Anisman, 1981). They may also underlie the anti-nociceptive and other behavioural consequences of stress. Therefore, before discussing these, it is useful to briefly outline some of the neurochemical consequences of aversive

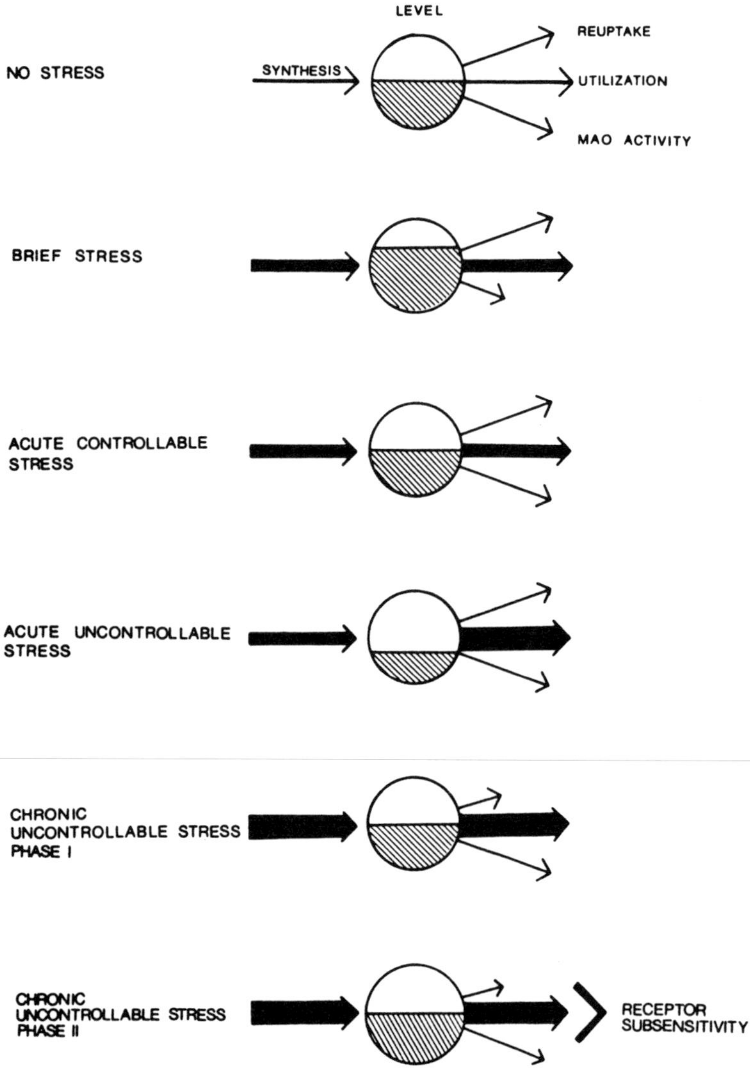

Figure 3.1 Schematic representation of changes of noradrenaline concentration, synthesis, utilization, reuptake and metabolism after brief stress, acute controllable and uncontrollable stress, and chronic uncontrollable stress (from Anisman and Zacharko, 1982).

stimulation. We have previously reviewed this area in some detail (e.g., Anisman, 1978; Sklar and Anisman, 1981; Anisman *et al.*, 1982; Anisman and Zacharko, 1982).

NEUROCHEMICAL CONSEQUENCES OF STRESS

There has been considerable interest, particularly during the last few years, in the effects of physical and psychological stressors on central and peripheral neurochemistry. Studies on laboratory animals have involved many stressors, including electric shock, restraint (immobilization), cold exposure, swimming, forced exercise, rotation, fumes, cutaneous irritants, and limb ischaemia. In humans, where only peripheral indices of neurotransmittter activity are readily monitored, stressors ranging from surgery, physical exercise and problem-solving tasks to prolonged space flight have been assessed (see the papers in Usdin *et al.*, 1976, 1980; see also Stone, 1975; Anisman *et al.*, 1982). To a large degree the findings are in agreement, although it should be remembered that factors such as stress severity and duration as well as the nature of the subject and its previous experience will influence the magnitude of neurochemical changes.

Greater attention has been devoted to the analysis of the effects of stress on noradrenaline than on other neurotransmitters and this is reflected in the present review. However, it should not be assumed that this transmitter is necessarily more important than others in subserving the behavioural consequences of stress. Also, the limited attention devoted to hormones, steroids and endogenous opiods, only reflects the fact that other contributors to this volume have considered them in some detail.

NORADRENALINE

Stress increases the synthesis and utilization of brain noradrenaline (Thierry *et al.*, 1971; Thierry, 1973). This has been noted in the hypothalamus, hippocampus, cortex, locus coeruleus, and amygdala (Korf *et al.*, 1973; Kvetnansky *et al.*, 1977; Nakagawa *et al.*, 1981). Soon after stress inception levels of noradrenaline may rise, possibly because of a transient inhibition of monoamine oxidase (Welch and Welch, 1970). The increased turnover and concentrations may reflect an adaptive change tending to maintain adequate supplies of the amine (see Figure 3.1).

If the stress is relatively severe or protracted, the rate of noradrenaline utilization increases still further, ultimately exceeding the rate of synthesis. Amine concentrations may then be reduced by up to 20–30% (see Stone, 1975; Weiss *et al.*, 1976; Anisman, 1978). Depletion varies not only with stress severity, but also with brain region (e.g., Nakagawa *et al.*, 1981). As depicted in Figure 3.2, both 60 and 180 footshocks (150 μA, 6 s duration) reduced

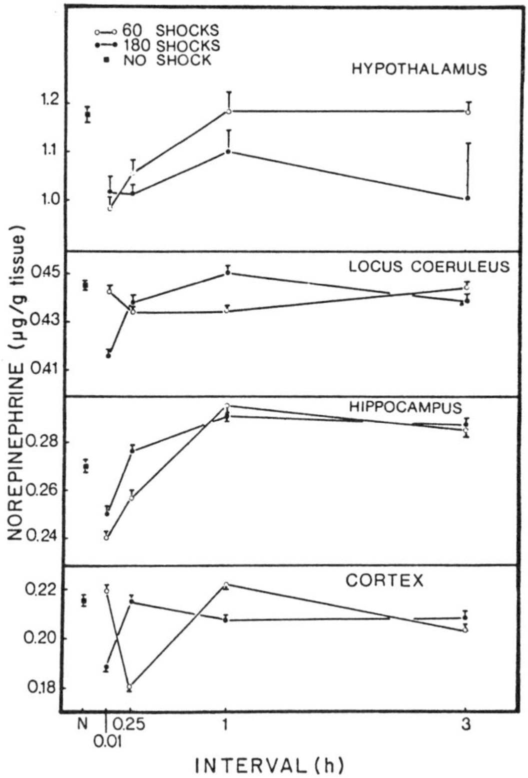

Figure 3.2 Brain regional noradrenaline concentrations (±s.e.m.) at various intervals after exposure to 60 or 180 inescapable shocks (6 s duration, 150 μA). Isolated squares denote concentrations for non-shocked mice. All differences noted in the text as significant are $p < 0.05$.

hypothalamic noradrenaline in mice. One hour after stress termination control values were reattained in mice that had received 60 shocks, whereas reduction of the amine persisted 3 h after 180 shocks.

Within the hypothalamus, noradrenaline reduction is marked in only certain nuclei, namely the ventromedial, supraoptic (Kvetnansky *et al.*, 1976), and the arcuate nuclei (Kobayashi *et al.*, 1976). Reductions have also been noted in other hypothalamic nuclei, including the paraventricular, dorsomedial and ventral premamillary nuclei as well as in the medial forebrain bundle while an increase was noted in the central dorsomedial nucleus (Kvetnansky *et al.*, 1976) but these changes were not statistically significant.

In agreement with others (Weiss *et al.*, 1981) we find that shock decreases noradrenaline in the locus coeruleus (and surrounding tissue including subcoeruleus and adjacent brainstem tissue). In contrast to the hypothalamic change, that in the locus coeruleus is marked after 180 but not 60 shocks, and reattains control levels within 1 h of stress termination. Using a substantially more severe stress regimen, Weiss *et al.* (1981) found that noradrenaline was reduced in the locus coeruleus and hypothalamus as long as 72 h and 48 h respectively after stress termination.

We find that the reductions of noradrenaline in hippocampus and cortex are less pronounced than in the hypothalamus and that more intense stress is required for this to occur. In Figure 3.2 both 60 and 180 shocks reduced hippocampal noradrenaline only by about 10% and basal concentrations were reattained within 15 min of 60 shocks and within 1 h of 180 shocks.

A fundamental factor in provoking the reduction of noradrenaline is the organism's ability to cope with the stressor. As observed by Weiss and his associates (Weiss *et al.*, 1976, 1981) and in our laboratory (Anisman *et al.*, 1980a) exposure to 60 escapable shocks did not reduce noradrenaline (see Figure 3.3). However, in mice that received an identical amount of shock in a yoked paradigm, it was appreciably reduced in hypothalamus and in hippocampus. In effect, not shock *per se* reduced noradrenaline, but rather the inability to control stress termination. We have proposed that when exposed to a stressor, animals seek behavioural means of coping and that this may be facilitated by the increased amine synthesis and utilization. When behavioural methods of coping are unavailable, or perceived as being unavailable, greater

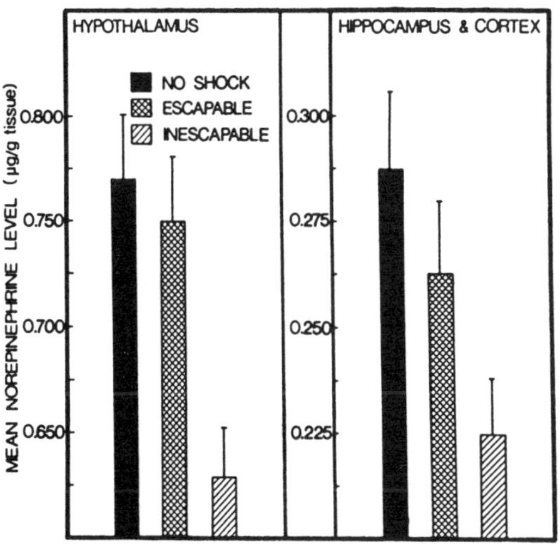

FIGURE 3.3 Brain regional noradrenaline concentrations (±s.e.m.) of mice that received no shock, 60 escapable shocks or yoked inescapable shock (from Anisman *et al.*, 1980a).

demands will be placed on endogenous neurochemical systems. Under these conditions, utilization of noradrenaline is more likely to exceed synthesis so that its concentration falls.

It should be noted that purely psychological stress may influence noradrenaline metabolism. For instance, it was recently reported (Iimori *et al.*, 1982) that exposure to the responses of other rats undergoing footshock resulted in increased noradrenaline utilization in the hypothalamus and amygdala and that its concentration was reduced in the latter region. Likewise, Welch and Welch (1968) reported that mere exposure to fighting by other mice reduced mouse brain noradrenaline. Also Stolk *et al.* (1974) found that the reductions seen soon after exposure to footshock were prevented if rats were permitted to fight during the shock session. Fighting conceivably served as a coping mechanism, thereby preventing the noradrenaline change even though shock continued to be applied.

Previous aversive stimulation may affect neurochemical responses to shock. As shown in Figure 3.4, the normal depletion of hypothalamic noradrenaline after a single session of 60 shocks is absent in mice that had previously had 14 sessions of 180 shocks on successive days (Bowers *et al.*, 1982). Moreover, we have consistently found that 24h after a chronic shock regimen, noradrenaline levels actually exceed basal values. In accordance with Thierry *et al.* (1968), we noted that exposure to chronic stress increases its utilization relative to that of both non-stressed and acutely stressed animals. Thus the above increse of noradrenaline was probably due to compensatory increase of synthesis. Indeed, Kobayashi *et al.* (1976) reported that tyrosine hydroxylase activity is increased after repeated stress exposure, while Kvetnansky *et al.* (1976) found that increases of noradrenaline during a single protracted session of immobilization was accompanied by increased dopamine-β-hydroxylase activity. Weiss *et al.* (1976) also reported that not only was noradrenaline synthesis increased after repeated stress but also its reuptake was inhibited, thus increasing the potential effectiveness of the released transmitter.

The fact that amine levels of chronically stressed animals approach those of control subjects should, of course, not be construed to imply that catecholamine activity has necessarily returned to normal. As depicted in Figure 3.1, amine turnover is substantially increased by chronic stress exposure. This may well have detrimental consequences as well as conceivably helping the animal to cope with the stressor. Further neuronal changes may also occur with chronic stress which tend to oppose the effects of the increase of release and blockade of reuptake of noradrenaline. Thus, following repeated exposure to a stressor, the sensitivity of noradrenaline β-receptors declines (Stone, 1979, 1980; Nomura *et al.*, 1981) and this down-regulation of postsynaptic receptors could moderate neuronal functioning.

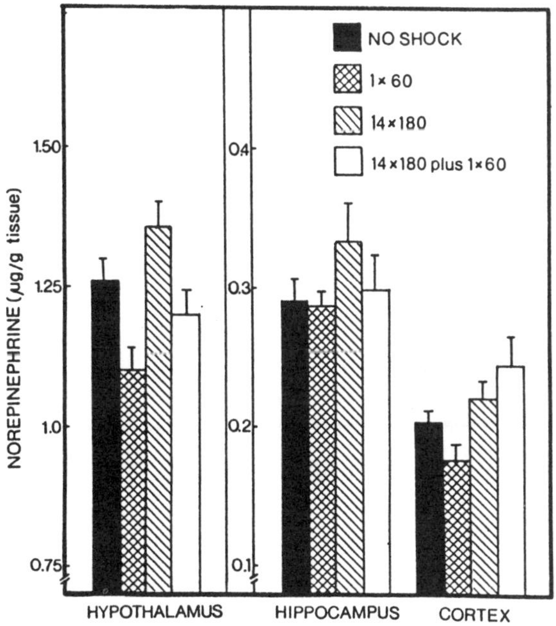

FIGURE 3.4 Brain regional noradrenaline concentrations (±s.e.m.) of mice that received no shock, a single session of 60 shocks, 14 sessions of 180 shocks, or 14 sessions of 180 shocks followed by a single session of 60 shocks. The 14 × 180 group were killed 24h after the last shock. The brains of the other groups were removed 1 min after the last shock.

Although reductions of noradrenaline concentration induced by stress are relatively transient, the mechanisms responsible for them may be subject to conditioning or sensitization and may thus have long-term repercussions. For instance, work in our laboratory (Anisman and Sklar, 1979) revealed that 24h after giving mice 60 footshocks (when noradrenaline levels and turnover are comparable to those of non-stressed animals) re-exposure to 10 shocks, which normally does not affect central noradrenaline concentrations, appreciably depleted it (see Figure 3.5). Thus, vulnerability to stress-provoked noradrenaline alterations is enhanced in previously stressed animals. Unpublished data from our laboratory indicates that the noradrenaline changes show cross-stressor sensitization effects, i.e., the depletion of noradrenaline provoked by uncontrollable footshock is more pronounced in mice that had previously been immersed in cold water than in naive mice (see Figure 3.6). Cassens *et al.* (1980) also find that a cue repeatedly paired with shock, upon subsequent presentation alone, increases the accumulation of the noradrenaline metabo-

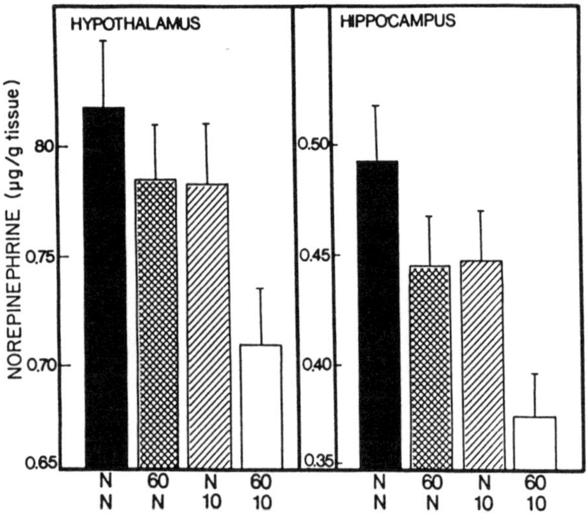

FIGURE 3.5 Brain regional noradrenaline concentrations (±s.e.m.) of mice that received no shock, 60 shocks followed 24 h later by no treatment, no treatment followed 24 h later by 10 shock trials, and 60 shocks followed 24 h later by 10 shocks.

lite, 3-methoxy-4-hydroxyphenylglycol sulphate (MHPG). Thus, the anticipation of shock may be sufficient to enhance noradrenaline metabolism.

In addition to stress controllability and duration, other factors affect the noradrenaline alterations provoked by stress. For example, the time of day during which mice are stressed influences the extent of noradrenaline depletion (Irwin *et al.*, 1982). As seen in Figure 3.7, between 0830 and 1000 and between 1300 and 1430 definite depletions of noradrenaline are provoked by both 60 and 180 shock presentations in the hypothalamus, locus coeruleus, and to a lesser extent in the hippocampus. However, between 1730 and 1900 hours the hypothalamic depletion is less pronounced and the locus coeruleus and hippocampus are not depleted. One possibility is that vulnerability to noradrenaline depletion is related to circadian variations in its turnover.

Housing conditions also influence the extent of noradrenaline alteration induced by stressors. It is well-established that individual and group housing have differential effects on its turnover in brain (Welch and Welch, 1970; Modigh, 1976). Moreover, young mice housed in isolation exhibit noradrenaline depletion more readily than group housed mice (Anisman and Sklar, 1981). Similarly, strains of mice not only differ in basal rates of noradrenaline turnover but are also differentially susceptible to noradrenaline reductions provoked by stress (e.g., Wimer *et al.*, 1973; see discussion in Anisman, 1978). Finally, it has been demonstrated that stress-induced reductions of noradrena-

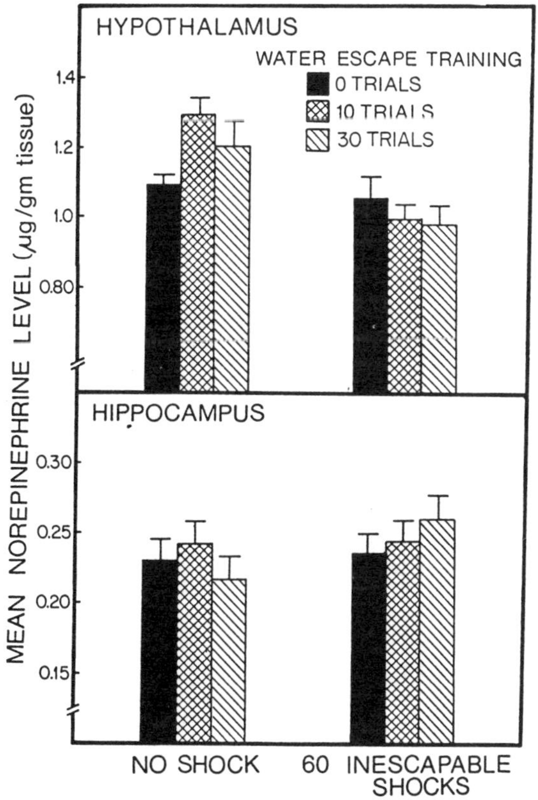

Figure 3.6 Brain regional noradrenaline concentrations (±s.e.m.) of mice that received 0, 10, or 30 water escape trials (15 °C) followed 24 h later by no treatment or 60 inescapable shocks.

line are more marked and persistent in older (18 months) than in younger (3 months) rats (Ritter and Pelzer, 1978).

Taken together, it seems that several variables interact to determine the magnitude of noradrenaline alterations engendered by stress. Some of these variables also influence the course of pathological states in which noradrenaline may be a contributing or modifying factor (see Sklar and Anisman, 1981). It may well be that behavioural changes elicited by uncontrollable stressors are also influenced by the above variables.

ADRENALINE

Owing to the low concentrations of adrenaline in brain, the study of the effects of stress on this amine awaited the development of sensitive assay procedures.

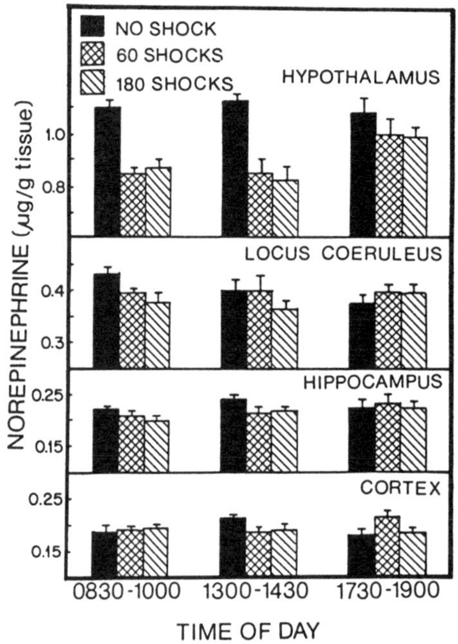

Figure 3.7 Brain regional noradrenaline concentrations (±s.e.m.) after exposure to 0, 60, or 180 shocks at different times of day.

Although only limited data are available, it does appear that stressors influence concentrations of adrenaline and the activity of the enzyme phenylethanolamine-*N*-methyltransferase which is required for its synthesis. For instance, acute immobilization stress (150min) decreased the activity of this enzyme in the locus coeruleus and nucleus tractus solitarius. After immobilization stress applied on successive days, the activity rose and approached control values (Saavedra, 1980). These results, it will be noted, are not paralleled by alterations of enzymes required for noradrenaline synthesis as this is increased by chronic stress.

As in the case of noradrenaline as little as 20 min of immobilization was sufficient to reduce adrenaline concentrations in the anterior hypothalamus and nucleus commisuralis, while concentrations were increased in the median eminence. With more prolonged immobilization (240min), adrenaline was decreased in the anterior hypothalamus, paraventricular and ventromedial nuclei, nucleus tractus solitarius, nucleus commisuralis and in the A1 and A2 regions (Saavedra *et al.*, 1979; Saavedra, 1980). The relationships of such alterations to factors such as stress controllability and their behavioural consequences have yet to be determined. It is likely that the adrenaline changes have peripheral repercussions, such as hypertensive effects (see Saavedra, 1980), which may in turn have behavioural consequences, particularly in paradigms involving aversive stimulation.

DOPAMINE

Despite early reports suggesting that stressors had little effect on dopamine, more recent evidence indicates fairly profound effects on this amine. However, alterations have not been noted in whole hypothalamus or in dopamine rich regions such as the substantia nigra. It seems that unlike the widespread noradrenaline changes induced by stressors those of dopamine are fairly restricted. Within the hypothalamus it only appears to be reduced in the arcuate nucleus (Kobayashi *et al.*, 1976; Kvetnansky *et al.*, 1976). However, the role of this nucleus in the secretion of hormones from the pituitary suggests that these DA changes could be involved in numerous behavioural consequences of stress, including antinociception.

Stressors can also provoke increased breakdown of the amine in the nucleus accumbens and in the mesolimbic frontal cortex, and may reduce dopamine concentration in the latter regions (Thierry *et al.*, 1976; Fadda *et al.*, 1978; Tissari *et al.*, 1979; Blanc *et al.*, 1980; Fekete *et al.*, 1981).

Although the role of coping factors in the above changes has not been determined, controllable and uncontrollable stress may differentially influence dopamine receptor sensitivity. Thus, Cherek *et al.* (1980) found that in the mesolimbic frontal cortex, 8 h uncontrollable shock over 4 days increased the sensitivity of low affinity dopamine receptors relative to that of rats that received controllable shock. Either coping factors (or enhanced perceived severity of the stress in the absence of coping) may have influenced the receptor changes.

As in the case of noradrenaline, it appears that dopamine alterations may be subject to conditioning or sensitization. For instance, Herman *et al.* (1981) who found that footshock increased dopamine metabolism in the mediofrontal and sulcal cortices, the nucleus accumbens and the amygdala also showed that simply placing rats in an environment previously associated with shock increased dopamine metabolism in the mediofrontal cortex. Likewise, Burns *et al.* (1981) found that a tone that had previously been paired with shock in a conditioned emotional response (CER) paradigm increased dopamine turnover in several brain regions. It therefore appears susceptible to threat or anticipation of a stressor as well as to the stressor itself. Thus, psychological factors may be important in governing dopamine alterations associated with aversive events.

SEROTONIN

As in the case of catecholamines, the turnover of serotonin has been shown to increase upon exposure to an aversive stimulus. Also after mild stress, levels of the amine may be increased (Welch and Welch, 1970) though a decrease may be evident after more intensive stress. It appears that the serotonin changes do not occur as readily as those of noradrenaline (Thierry, 1973). It was reported that 150 min of immobilization increased serotonin concentrations in several hypothalamic nuclei (Culman *et al.*, 1980), but 3 h of immobilization resulted in 5HT reductions in cingulate cortex, median eminence, supra-chiasmatic nucleus, amygdala, and dorsal raphé (Palkovits *et al.*, 1976).

The contribution of coping factors to the serotonin changes has been examined by several investigators. Petty and Sherman (1982) reported that escapable shock increased serotonin concentrations in the anterior cortex, whereas yoked inescapable shock reduced them in the septum and anterior cortex. Moreover, the reduction was evident as long as 5 days later. Weiss *et al.* (1981) likewise reported that uncontrollable shock decreased serotonin concentrations in the locus coeruleus but not in the remainder of the brainstem, while escapable shock had no effect. They suggested that the noradrenaline alterations induced by uncontrollable and controllable shock reflect the relative stressfulnes of these procedures, whereas the serotonin changes reflect the behavioural response to the stressors.

ACETYLCHOLINE

Different aversive stimuli have been found to influence brain acetylcholine the alterations varying with brain region and severity of the stressor. For instance, 20–25 min after cold exposure for 1 h, acetylcholine turnover was reduced in the frontal cortex but not following 4 or 24 h of such treatment. In hypothalamus, however, both 1 and 23 h of cold exposure reduced acetylcholine turnover (Costa *et al.*, 1980).

Zajaczkowska (1975) reported that soon after stress inception, a transient decrease of the transmitter was evident, followed within 40 min by an increase. Increased acetylcholine concentrations induced by a stressor may be related to the animal's ability to cope with the aversive stimulus. In two separate experiments, Karczmar *et al.* (1973) reported that acetylcholine was increased by unavoidable shock, but not by avoidable shock. Furthermore, Cherek *et al.* (1980) found that increased muscarinic receptor binding was evident afer uncontrollable shock applied on five consecutive days but not after escapable shock. Finally, cholinergic changes induced by stressors (like those of other transmitters) respond to conditioning or sensitization as exposure to a cue that had previously been paired with shock caused increased acetylcholine concentrations (Hingtgen *et al.*, 1976).

OPIATE PEPTIDES

Endorphins and adrenocorticotrophic hormone (ACTH) are present within the same secretory granules of the pituitary (Guillemin *et al.*, 1977; Weber *et al.*, 1978) as well as in brain (Watson *et al.*, 1978; Krieger *et al.*, 1979). Moreover, environmental stressors (long known to stimulate ACTH secretion), also stimulate secretion of endorphin from the pituitary and thus increase plasma concentrations of the endogenous opioid (Blasig *et al.*, 1978; Santagostino *et al.*, 1978; Baizman *et al.*, 1979). Stressors are also reported to either increase (Madden *et al.*, 1977; Akil *et al.*, 1978) or decrease (Rossier *et al.*, 1978) endorphin concentration in whole brain or in hypothalamus under various conditions.

A fairly extensive analysis by Barta and Yashpal (1981) has revealed that severity and duration of stress influence endorphin changes, and that these changes vary with brain region. After acute swimming stress (20°C, 3 min) endorphins decreased in the intermediate, posterior and anterior lobes of the pituitary while increased levels were evident in the paraventricular nucleus, nucleus interstitialis, striae terminalis, central amygdaloid nucleus, and dorsal raphé nucleus. More severe swimming conditions (4°C, 3 min) caused more pronounced increases. With the milder stress procedure (but not with the more severe procedure) the endorphin changes were no longer evident after 21 swim sessions. Thus, adaptation to the effects of a stressor may occur on its repeated application but the course of the adaptation appears to depend upon severity. Whether psychological variables known to influence catecholamine activity also influence endorphin activity requires further investigation, although data suggests that stress controllability may be a determinant of opioid changes (see Jackson *et al.*, 1979) and endorphin changes induced by stress can be reinduced by cues that had been associated with it (Chance *et al.*, 1978; DeVries *et al.*, 1979).

BEHAVIOURAL DEFICITS INDUCED BY STRESSORS

Escape performance

The effects of physical and psychological insults on numerous behaviours have been examined. In at least some cases it appears that the behavioural outcomes are related to the controllability of the initial stress. For example, it is well established that escape behaviour is not adversely affected by prior exposure to controllable (escapable) shock but that exposure to an equivalent amount of uncontrollable (yoked) shock causes severe deficits of later escape performance (see reviews in Maier and Seligman, 1976; Weiss *et al.*, 1979; Anisman *et al.*, 1981a). Several mechanisms have been suggested for this. According to a cognitive explanation advanced by Maier and Seligman (1976), animals learn during inescapable shock that their responses are ineffective in terminating the aversive stimulation, i.e. that they are 'helpless'. Accordingly, when subsequently exposed to escapable stressors, these animals do not attempt to escape. Maier and Seligman (1976) also proposed that uncontrollable stressors induce emotional and motivational changes and disturb the learning of novel response-outcome associations. More recently, Maier and Jackson (1979) raised the possibility that the anti-nociception associated with uncontrollable shock may also contribute to the defective performance of tasks involving aversive motivation.

Escape deficits induced by uncontrollable shock have also been related to the neurochemical concomitants of the stress. In particular, it has been argued that the noradrenaline changes are responsible for the behavioural disturbances (e.g. Anisman *et al.*, 1979a; Weiss *et al.*, 1976, 1981). Anisman *et al.* (1979a,b, 1981a,b) also suggested that reduction of dopamine and increase of acetylcholine concentrations contribute to the behavioural disruption. It was proposed that these neurochemical changes cause defects in the initiation of responses to weak stimuli (e.g., a conditioned stimulus), and difficulties in maintaining responses to strong stimuli (e.g., shock). Indeed, using a typical shuttle escape task, deficits are not evident in mice or rats after uncontrollable shock. If, however, they are required to run from one compartment to the next and then back again to escape shock then pronounced escape deficits are evident (Maier *et al.*, 1973; Maier and Testa, 1975). These investigators maintained that because running is high in the rodent's defensive repertoire, the cognitive consequences induced by inescapable shock are masked in a simple shuttle escape task but when the task is associatively more difficult (namely the shuttle procedure), then cognitive consequences of uncontrollable shock cause a performance deficit. The shuttle procedure, however, is not only more associatively difficult but may be motorically more demanding as even rats that had not been exposed to inescapable shock needed 5–10 s for an escape response. Thus defective escape may have become manifest simply because the task involved impaired response maintenance induced by inescapable shock.

A series of experiments in our laboratory (Anisman *et al.*, 1978) indicated that activity during shock declined rapidly both during and between shock presentations. Mice previously exposed to inescapable shock showed more rapid declines than mice that had previously received escapable shock. At the onset of each shock presentation, relatively high activities were evident in all groups. It was suggested that these favoured adequate performance when escape was possible at the time of shock onset irrespective of previous shock experience. Conversely, the decline of shock-elicited activity after several seconds would favour inadequate escape performance, especially in mice previously exposed to inescapable shock.

In order to evaluate this possibility, the effects of inescapable shock on escape performance were assessed in an experiment in which mice were required to sustain an active response for various times before escape was possible. Following inescapable shock (60 shocks, 6 s duration, 150 μA) mice were tested in a shuttle escape task. Escape was possible immediately or 2, 4, or 6 s after shock onset. Thus, the same response was required of each group in

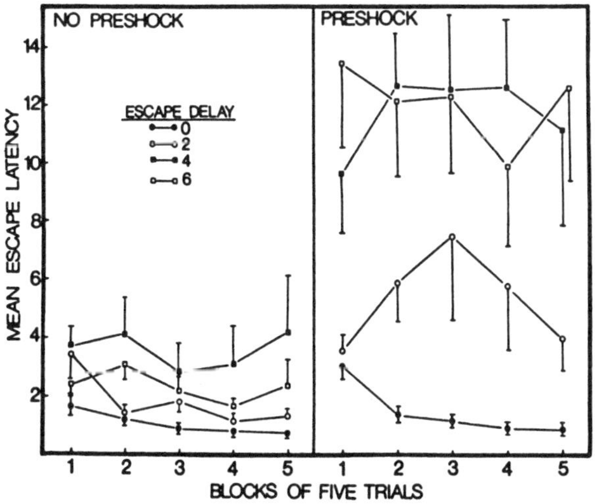

FIGURE 3.8 Mean (±s.e.m.) escape latencies 24h after exposure to no shocks or to 60 shocks of 6s duration. Escape was possible 0, 2, 4, or 6s after shock onset (from Anisman *et al.*, 1978).

order to escape, but the duration during which it was sustained differed between groups. As depicted in Figure 3.8, previous inescapable shock did not affect escape upon shock onset but it did impair escape when 4–6s active response was required. It should be emphasized that we find that similar but escapable shock does not influence later escape behaviour.

The disruptive effects of inescapable shock are not restricted to tests involving escape from shock, but are also evident in tasks involving other aversive stimuli. For example, Irwin *et al.* (1980) reported that inescapable shock disrupts later performance in a water escape task. Moreover, these deficits were dependent on the degree to which the test situation provoked motor difficulties. For example, as seen in Figure 3.9, inescapable shock did not influence escape performance from water at 20°C but it did impair escape in colder water (15°C), where difficulties of response maintenance were more acute. Thus, despite the increased motivation to escape which is presumably induced by the colder water, the associated motor consequences reveal the effects of the inescapable shock. In still colder water (10°C) performance of all animals is impaired irrespective of previous shock and differences between naive and inescapably shocked mice were no longer apparent.

Additional evidence consistent with response maintenance deficits being responsible for interference with escape is that levels of shock-elicited activity predict later escape behaviour (Anisman *et al.*, 1979b). Furthermore, altering shock-elicited activity alters escape performance. Thus, the superimposition of a startle stimulus increased shock-elicited activity and eliminated the escape deficits provoked by inescapable shock (Anisman *et al.*, 1978).

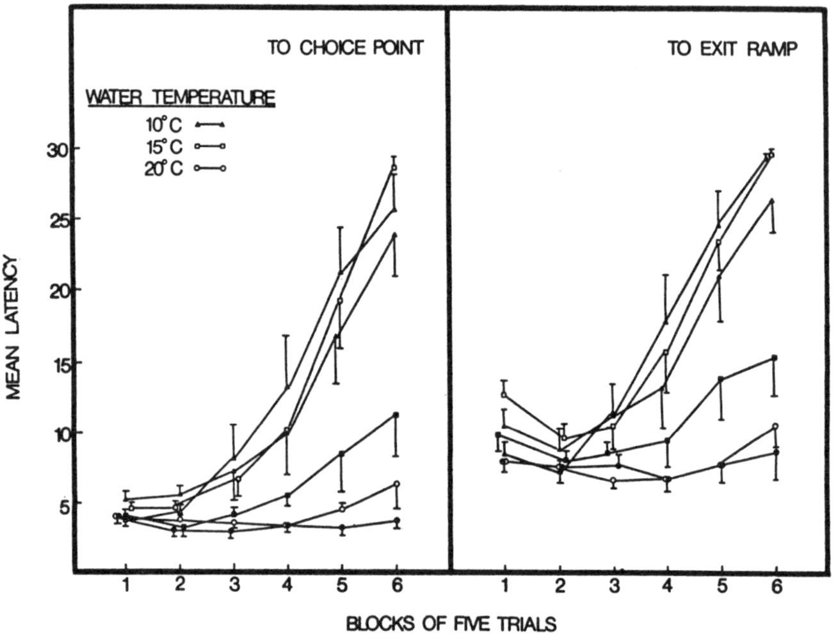

FIGURE 3.9 Mean (±s.e.m.) latency to swim to the choice point and escape ramp of a water-maze (10 °C, 15 °C, or 20 °C) by mice that received no shock or 60 inescapable shocks 24 h earlier (from Irwin *et al.*, 1980).

Several correlational analyses support a neurochemical mechanism for the escape deficits. It will be recalled that noradrenaline is depleted by a single session but not by repeated sessions of inescapable shock (Weiss *et al.*, 1976). These investigators also found that the increase of noradrenaline on repeated shock was accompanied by improved escape performance. Of course, these data do not prove a causal relationship between the increase of noradrenaline and escape behaviour, but they do challenge purely cognitive interpretations which would predict that escape would become more rather than less impaired with repeated stress application.

The effects of various drugs on escape deficits are consistent with their mediation by catecholaminergic and cholinergic changes as we showed that the tyrosine hydroxylase inhibitor, α-methyl-*p*-tyrosine, the dopamine-β-hydroxylase inhibitor, FLA-63, the dopamine receptor blockers, haloperidol and pimozide, and the cholinesterase inhibitor, physostigmine (like inescapable shock) markedly reduced shock-elicited activity (Anisman *et al.*, 1979a, 1981b). Moreover, as depicted in Figure 3.10, these compounds also disrupted escape performance when mice were required to sustain an active response for several seconds before escape was possible. Figure 3.10 shows results with α-methyl-*p*-tyrosine, FLA-63 and pimozide. The same pattern was evident

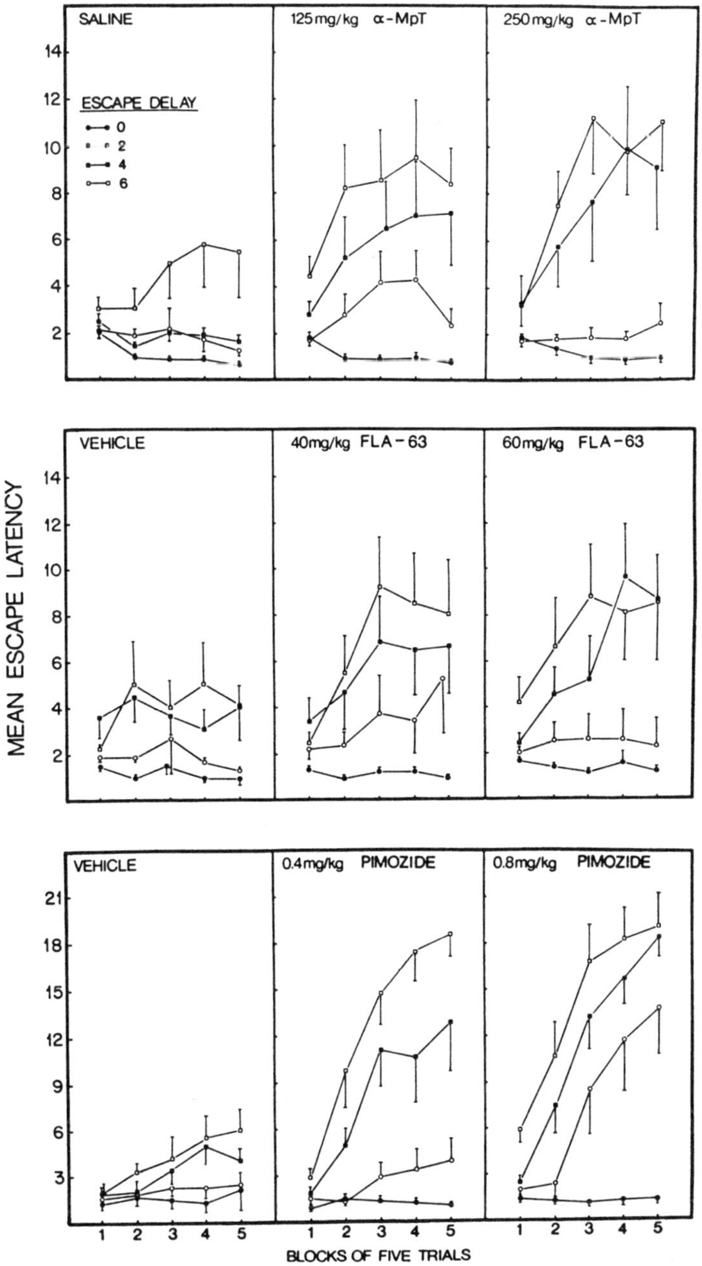

Figure 3.10 Mean (±s.e.m.) escape latencies of mice treated with α-methyl-*p*-tyrosine, FLA-63 or pimozide. Escape was possible 0, 2, 4, or 6s after shock onset (from Anisman *et al.*, 1979a).

using haloperidol and physostigmine. Clearly, depleting catecholamines, blocking DA receptors, or increasing ACh provoke behavioural disturbances which parallel those induced by inescapable shock. The fact that all of these treatments lead to behavioural disturbances should not be construed to imply a completely non-specific mechanism. For example, lithium at doses that provoke taste aversion did not induce escape deficits. Likewise, neither increasing 5-hydroxytryptamine concentrations by treating mice with 5-hydroxytryptophan plus MK-486, nor decreasing them by treatment with *p*-chlorophenylalanine influenced escape behaviour. Furthermore, we have recently observed that 75 mg/kg of DSP-4, which reduced hippocampal and cortical noradrenaline by up to 70% but only moderately reduced hypothalamic values, did not influence escape performance. The latter result, incidentally, suggests that hippocampal and cortical noradrenaline changes do not affect escape performance.

In agreement with our data, it has been reported (Weiss *et al.*, 1979) that catecholamine depletion induced by the neurotoxin, 6-hydroxydopamine, severely disrupted escape performance in a shuttle and wheel-turning task which imposed strenuous motor demands. In contrast, the depletion did not influence escape when rats were required to make a nose-poke response which involved little motor difficulty. Similarly, Glazer and Weiss (1976) found that the deficits of escape performance induced by uncontrollable shock, were pronounced with a shuttle-escape task but absent with the nose-poke task. Here again, it seems that the effects of drug treatments depended on the motor demands placed on the animal.

Parallel effects of inescapable shock and drug-induced escape deficits were also observed when mice received escape training prior to the drug or inescapable shock experience. It is well documented that previous training in an escape task prevents the deficits of escape performance ordinarily provoked by inescapable shock (see Maier and Seligman, 1976). We have similarly found that drug induced escape deficits are not evident or are minimized in mice previously trained to escape (Anisman *et al.*, 1979a). Figure 3.11 shows that the escape deficits ordinarily induced by haloperidol at moderate doses are decreased if mice previously received 10 or 30 escape trials. We have recently also found that deficits of water escape performance similar to those induced by inescapable shock can be provoked by pimozide and that this effect is reduced if mice are previously trained to escape (Corradini *et al.*, 1982).

While catecholamine antagonists mimic the disruptive effects of inescapable shock, catecholamine stimulants (and anticholinergics) eliminate the performance deficits due to inescapable shock. The effects of L-dopa administered prior to escape testing of naive mice and mice previously exposed to inescapable shock is shown in Figure 3.12. Clearly, the escape deficits were eliminated by the drug (Anisman *et al.*, 1979a). We have observed the same effects using the dopamine agonist apomorphine and the noradrenaline

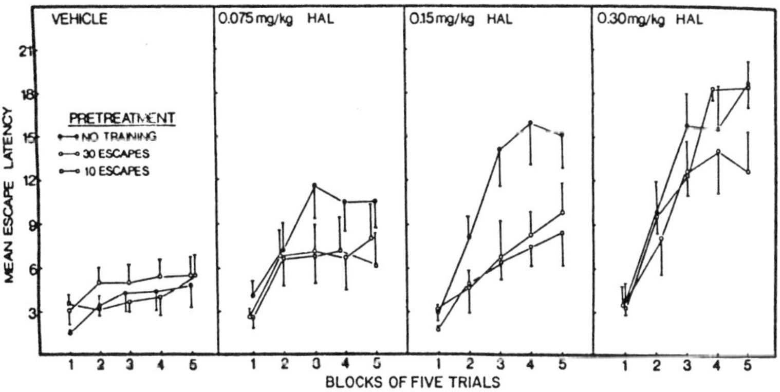

FIGURE 3.11 Mean (±s.e.m.) escape latencies of mice treated with various doses of haloperidol. Twenty-four hours earlier mice had received 0, 10, or 30 trials of escape training (from Anisman *et al.*, 1979a).

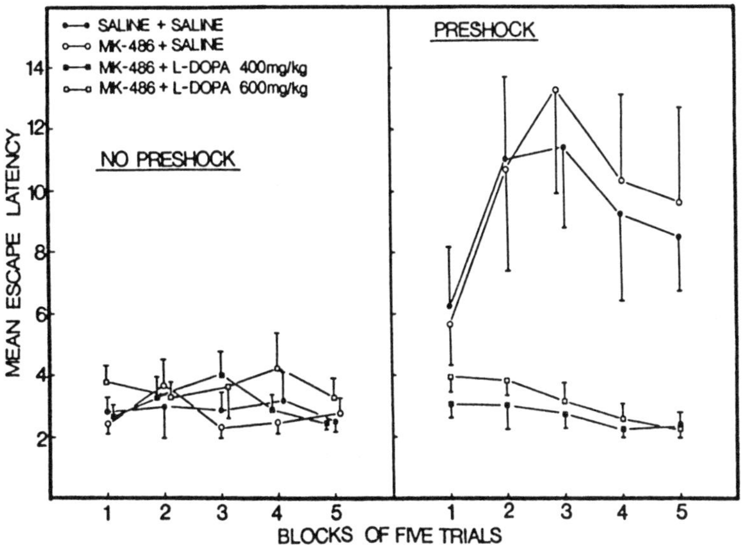

FIGURE 3.12 Mean (±s.e.m.) escape latencies of mice exposed to 0 or 60 inescapable shocks 24h earlier. Prior to testing mice were treated wtih MK486 + L-dopa or vehicle (adapted from Anisman *et al.*, 1979a).

agonist, clonidine (Anisman *et al.*, 1980b). These agents also prevented the escape deficits when given before inescapable shock. In addition, treatments known to act as effective antidepressants, such as repeated administration of nortriptyline or desmethylimipramine (Sherman and Petty, 1980; Telner and Singhal, 1981) effectively antagonized the behavioural disturbances induced by inescapable shock. Finally, when administered prior to escape training, the anticholinergic drug, scopolamine eliminates the influence of previous inescapable shock (Anisman *et al.*, 1981b). In contrast to catecholamine stimulants however, scopolamine was ineffective as a prophylactic. Thus, although the effects of the various above drug treatments are similar they are not identical. As indicated by Sherman and Petty (1980) it is possible that the induction and maintenance of the effects of inescapable shock on subsequent escape may involve independent mechanisms.

While the pharmacological experiments described agree with a neurochemical mechanism for the above effect, they do not necessarily exclude cognitive factors as treatments which reduce catecholamine activity might provoke 'helplessness' and in turn promote the effect of inescapable shock. Conversely, treatments that increase catecholamine functioning could have opposing actions. However, as cognitive changes can only be reliably measured in man, it is perhaps more parsimonious to consider the behavioural deficits in terms of neurochemical changes.

Associative factors

Although we have emphasized the role of motor changes in response to inescapable shock, other effects might also contribute to the escape deficits. In accordance with the suggestions of Maier and Seligman (1976) experiments by Jackson *et al.* (1980) revealed that following inescapable shock, rats were unable to acquire a response-choice discrimination response as readily as non-shocked animals. These investigators argued that although inescapable shock does not influence cue-shock associations, such a treatment will disrupt the acquisition of response-choice associations. Experiments in our laboratory, however, have not confirmed these findings. In water escape experiments (Irwin *et al.*, 1980) the escape deficits induced by inescapable shock were not accompanied by disruption of a position discrimination, nor was reversal of a position discrimination affected by the shock treatment. In more recent, as yet unpublished experiments, in which performance was assessed using a discriminated Y-maze shock escape task, it was found that inescapable shock did not influence later acquisition of a cue discrimination response or a response-choice discrimination (i.e., in a task in which the safe arm of one trial is the shock arm of the next trial so that external stimuli are not cues for appropriate responding). Likewise, inescapable shock did not influence discrimination performance by mice previously trained in these tasks.

In contrast to these findings, uncontrollable shock was found to influence performance in a reversal learning task (Anisman and Zacharko, unpublished). In particular, following acquisition of a response-choice, mice exhibited negative transference when required to perform the response opposite to that which previously proved successful. With continued testing, mice acquired the reversal response. Mice exposed to inescapable shock after initial response-choice acquisition showed negative transference in the reversal task, indicating that the retention of the initially established response was unimpaired. Unlike mice that had not been exposed to inescapable shock, these animals failed to acquire the reversal response, but persisted in the response that had previously proved successful. Uncontrollable shock may not only narrow the organism's defensive repertoire, but may also influence response selection patterns. Thus, mice exposed to inescapable shock persist in utilizing response patterns that were previously well entrenched but are now inappropriate. This perseverative pattern of responding may be interpreted as an associative deficit.

In yet another series of experiments (Bruto and Anisman, 1981) we determined whether uncontrollable shock influenced exploratory behaviour in a free-running radial (8-arm) maze. Normal mice exhibit alternation behaviour (i.e., they entered those arms least recently visited). Moreover, they frequently visited immediately adjacent arms (adjacent alternation). A single session of inescapable shock which produced deficits in a shuttle or water swim task had only moderate effects on this behaviour, i.e. the rate of *adjacent* alternation was specifically reduced so that although the rate of alternation remained high, its pattern appeared less organized. It is likely that this resulted from attentional deficits rather than from associative disturbances.

Anti-nociception and escape behaviour

As in the case of the escape deficits, it appears that escapable and inescapable shock differentially influence performance in tests of analgesia. In both a hot-plate and tail-flick test, only inescapable shock increased response latencies (Jackson *et al.*, 1979). Moreover, although the analgesia was relatively transient, it was re-established on re-exposure to a few shock presentations. On the basis of such findings, Maier and Jackson (1979) suggested that the anti-nociceptive effects of uncontrollable shock may contribute to deficits of escape behaviour. Indeed, experiments by Maier and his associates (Jackson *et al.*, 1979; Maier *et al.*, 1980; Moye *et al.*, 1981; Maier *et al.*, 1982) revealed that several variables that influence escape performance after inescapable shock also modify the anti-nociceptive reaction. Of course, these parallel effects do not prove a causal relationship between anti-nociception and escape performance and indeed, there is evidence that the relationship is simply a correlational one.

Experiments in our laboratory (Mah *et al.*, 1980) indicated that shock controllability is not necessarily essential for the provocation of the anti-nociception. Exposure to 15 escapable or inescapable shock trials both induced anti-nociception. This diminished with further shock presentation, so that 60 escapable shocks produced only a modest anti-nociception, while it was entirely absent after 60 uncontrollable shocks. Other investigators have likewise found that a biphasic analgesic response occurs as a function of the number of shocks animals receive. For instance, Grau *et al.* (1981) reported that analgesia occurs following 20 shock presentations, is absent after 40 shocks, and then reappears after 60–80 shocks. Furthermore, work by other investigators (Lewis *et al.*, 1980, 1981), has indicated the existence of two forms of analgesia. Analgesia could be induced by brief continuous shock or by more protracted intermittent shock but only the latter was reversible by naloxone and cross-tolerant with morphine-induced analgesia (see also Maier *et al.*, 1980; Grau *et al.*, 1981; Drugan *et al.*, 1981). In effect, it seems that two biochemically distinct forms of analgesia exist, one, induced by relatively protracted stress, appears to be opioid mediated. The other is induced by briefer shock and mediated by non-opioid mechanisms. It is conceivable that the difference between our results and those of Maier's laboratory on the role of controllability in the induction of analgesia stems from the number of shock trials employed. None the less, our data question the role of analgesia in the induction of the escape interference as the number of shocks (60) necessary to produce catecholamine changes in brain and escape deficits was the same as that after which analgesia was no longer present. The independence of the analgesia and escape deficits is further indicated by the lack of effect of analgesic doses of morphine sulphate (10–30 mg/kg) on escape behaviour (Mah *et al.*, 1980, Table 3.1). Also, we find that treatment with naloxone before escape training does not antagonize the escape interference engendered by inescapable shock.

It will be recalled that upon stress inception, the turnovers of catecholamines and 5-hydroxytryptamine are increased. Initially, amine levels increase but as the aversive stimulation continues they decline. The initial anti-nociception

TABLE 3.1. Effects of morphine on paw-lick hot-plate escape and shuttle escape latencies of mice.

	Latency (s)			
		Morphine (mg/kg)		
Test	Saline ($n = 10$)	10.0 ($n = 10$)	20.0 ($n = 10$)	30.0 ($n = 10$)
Paw-lick	13.80 ± 2.18	37.10 ± 5.05*	53.83 ± 2.96*	55.60 ± 3.15*
Hot-plate escape	10.89 ± 1.51	26.60 ± 6.32*	39.79 ± 6.46*	54.04 ± 3.66*
Shuttle-escape	2.62 ± 0.43	2.86 ± 0.64	3.29 ± 0.49	3.00 ± 0.43

Values are means ± s.e.m.
*$p < 0.05$ relative to saline-treated mice.
From Mah *et al.* (1980).

(i.e., after limited shock) is associated with increased amine turnover and levels. Therefore, the initial short-term anti-nociception might have reflected a transient adaptive response to stress mediated by the initial increase of catecholamine activity. Alternatively, it may merely have reflected increased reactivity to environmental stimuli, so that the aversiveness of stimulation appeared to be reduced (i.e. heightened activity may interfere with responses such as paw-lick). We therefore studied the effects of various catecholamine stimulants and antagonists on tail-flick and paw-lick latencies (Bruto and Anisman, unpublished). As shown in Table 3.2, catecholamine stimulants markedly increased both response latencies.

Drugs which reduced catecholamine levels or blocked their receptors decreased response latencies but these effects were considerably less marked than those of stimulants. These data may indicate that the anti-nociception induced by a relatively small number of shocks may be directly related to catecholamine and 5HT release. However, it is also possible that the reduced responsiveness was not due to genuine analgesia, but resulted from alteration of some other behaviour. For example, the catecholamine stimulants may have increased paw-lick latencies simply because animals were more active, so that they had less 'opportunity' to paw-lick, or even spent less time in contact with the hot-plate. However, these factors are less likely to influence tail-flick latencies.

We do not dismiss the possibility that release of endogenous opioids is responsible for the analgesic peak on continued stressful stimulation. Likewise, we do not question the role of stress controllability in the induction of the anti-nociception. The findings that stressors or associated cues induced endorphin release and analgesia and that the latter is reversed by naloxone, exhibits tolerance and is cross tolerant with morphine are certainly consistent with opioid mediated stress-induced anti-nociception. We do question, however, whether this anti-nociception is causally linked with the escape deficits caused by inescapable shock and we believe that its expression is vulnerable to the effects of stress unrelated to alterations of pain sensitivity. Finally, we raise the possibility that catecholamine alterations may also contribute to the second analgesia peak. After all, noradrenaline changes induced by stressors (like the anti-nociception) undergo adaptation with repeated stress, and are influenced by re-exposure to a stressor or cues associated with it. Moreover, endorphins may modulate catecholamine neurotransmission in some brain regions (Versteeg *et al.*, 1978). The above possibilities warrant further consideration.

Motivational consequences

Advocates of hypotheses of escape deficits based on either helplessness or neurochemistry have suggested that inescapable shock may result in motivational disturbances. Indeed, we have proposed that uncontrollable aversive

TABLE 3.2 Effects of drug treatments on paw-lick (48° and 52°) and tail-flick latencies.

		Paw-lick (48°)	Paw-lick (52°)	Tail-flick
Saline		21.62 ± 2.63		9.25 ± 0.59
L-dopa	100 mg/kg	28.87 ± 2.46*		—
	200 mg/kg	47.75 ± 4.75*		—
	400 mg/kg	57.25 ± 1.81*		15.62 ± 1.66*
Saline		14.80 ± 1.33	12.70 ± 1.78	10.32 ± 0.44
Pargyline	25 mg/kg	16.50 ± 0.98	9.10 ± 1.43	9.96 ± 0.88
	50 mg/kg	19.10 ± 1.67*	9.40 ± 0.99	8.60 ± 0.74
	100 mg/kg	21.50 ± 1.38*	10.30 ± 2.15	9.14 ± 0.56
Saline		25.33 ± 7.21	13.33 ± 2.33	11.16 ± 1.74
Desmethyl-imipramine	25 mg/kg	32.08 ± 3.46	17.83 ± 1.64	10.25 ± 0.64
	50 mg/kg	57.50 ± 2.50*	19.16 ± 0.83*	15.16 ± 1.16*
Saline			9.87 ± 1.57	8.12 ± 0.31
Apomorphine	0.25 mg/kg		—	7.43 ± 0.87
	0.50 mg/kg		14.12 ± 1.68*	8.56 ± 0.75
	1.00 mg/kg		16.06 ± 1.16*	8.00 ± 0.71
	1.50 mg/kg		18.00 ± 1.46*	8.37 ± 0.38
Saline		18.37 ± 1.96	10.12 ± 1.74	7.81 ± 1.11
Clonidine	0.25 mg/kg	33.50 ± 2.57	—	8.06 ± 0.57
	0.50 mg/kg	27.12 ± 2.48*	17.12 ± 1.90*	8.50 ± 1.52
	1.00 mg/kg	35.50 ± 5.37*	18.06 ± 1.72*	10.62 ± 2.13
	1.50 mg/kg	37.37 ± 5.11*	17.31 ± 1.56*	10.43 ± 2.12
Saline			11.68 ± 1.40	9.06 ± 1.48
Scopolamine	0.5 mg/kg		18.62 ± 0.90*	11.50 ± 0.95
	1.0 mg/kg		19.62 ± 0.37*	9.06 ± 1.60
	2.0 mg/kg		19.31 ± 0.47*	10.00 ± 2.61
Vehicle		16.00 ± 1.57		
Haloperidol	0.075 mg/kg	18.37 ± 2.63		
	0.15 mg/kg	19.00 ± 2.11		
	0.30 mg/kg	21.87 ± 2.84		
Vehicle + saline		17.50 ± 2.36		
Vehicle + apomorphine (1.00 mg/kg)		34.75 + 5.09*		
Haloperidol (0.30 mg/kg) + saline		19.12 ± 1.74		
Haloperidol + apomorphine		17.87 ± 1.71		
No shock		27.25 ± 2.83	13.12 ± 1.76	9.37 ± 0.53
15 shock		52.66 ± 3.98*	18.75 ± 0.81*	19.25 ± 0.52*
60 shock		43.25 ± 6.65*	17.62 ± 0.81*	9.93 ± 1.81
180 shock		—	14.25 ± 1.44	—

*$p < 0.05$ relative to non-drug animals.
From Bruto and Anisman (unpublished report).

events precipitate or aggravate clinical depression in humans (Anisman and Zacharko, 1982), and might conceivably have a role in one of the fundamental symptoms of depression, namely anhedonia. Unfortunately, it is not practical to assess motivational changes in escape paradigms, since performance will be affected by factors such as response initiation and maintenance. The usefulness of paradigms involving appetite motivation may also be limited owing to the need to impose food deprivation which may be a confounding variable.

In our experiments we assessed motivational/reinforcement processes by studying the effects of controllable and uncontrollable shock on intracranial self-stimulation. Accumulating evidence suggests that dopamine neuronal activity enhances self-stimulation (see Wise, 1978 for a review), though its role may not be of primary importance (Arbuthnott, 1980; Wise, 1980). Numerous brain regions rich in dopamine or through which dopamine pathways pass support self-stimulation (see German and Bowden, 1974; Wise, 1978 for reviews) and as previously stated, the effects of uncontrollable shock on dopamine activity varies with brain region. For example, it is altered in the nucleus accumbens and some regions of the hypothalamus but little change is evident in the substantia nigra. If uncontrollable shock affects motivational/ reinforcement processes then resultant changes of self-stimulation responding might also vary with the brain region. The following experiments were therefore done.

Following electrode placement in the medial forebrain bundle, nucleus accumbens or substantia nigra pars compacta, mice were trained to dip their head to obtain electrical brain stimulation. When stable rates of responding were obtained, mice were divided into three groups matched for baseline response and given 60 escapable shocks, yoked inescapable shock, or no shock. Immediately thereafter, and 24h and 168h later they were tested for self-stimulation for a ten minute period. Escapable shock did not alter rates of responding for brain stimulation of any of the brain regions examined (Figure 3.13).

In contrast, uncontrollable shock markedly reduced response rates when stimulating the nucleus accumbens and the medial forebrain bundle, but had little effect when the substantia nigra was stimulated. Changes in either general arousal, attentional processes, or motoric deficits might have been expected to lead to comparable reductions from all brain regions. Likewise, the reduction in responding for rewarding brain stimulation following inescapable shock is not rate specific since baseline rates of responding from the substantia nigra were comparable to those from the medial forebrain bundle. The reduced response rate from the nucleus accumbens but not from the substantia nigra is consistent with mediation by the region-specific alterations of dopamine activity. The reduced rate of responding in the case of the medial forebrain bundle could reflect altered dopamine activity either in the hypothalamus or in fibres of passage through it. Finally, the lack of

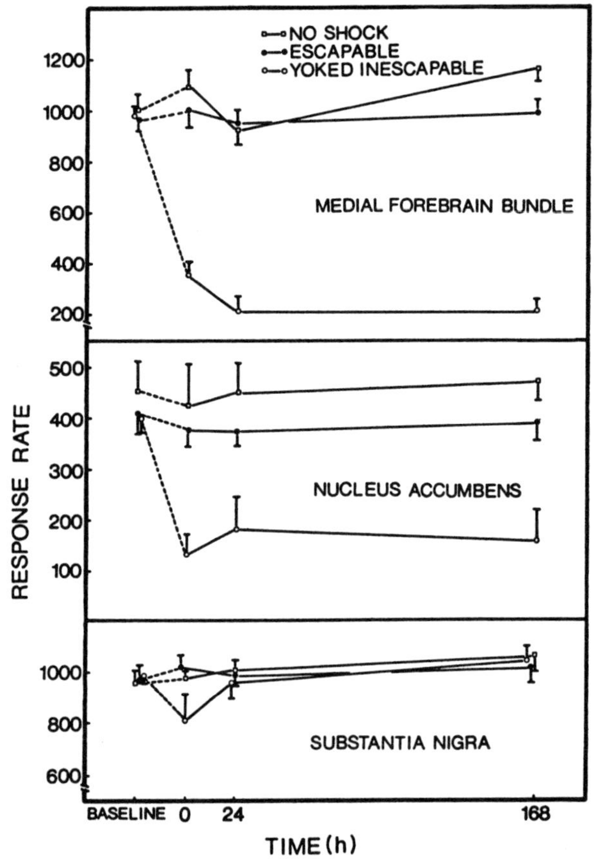

Figure 3.13 Mean (±s.e.m.) rate of responding for electrical brain stimulation of the medial forebrian bundle, nucleus accumbens, and substantia nigra of mice exposed to no shock, 60 escapable shocks, or yoked inescapable shocks. Baseline rates and rates 0, 24, or 168h after treatment are shown (from Zacharko *et al.*, 1982).

effect of escapable shock indicates that controllability of the shock rather than the shock *per se* was necessary for the response deficits to occur.

Taken together, these data are consistent with effects of uncontrollable aversive events on motivational/reinforcement processes in paradigms involving positive reinforcement. Whether motivational changes induced by stressors influence performance in escape paradigms is not known, nor is it known whether the anti-nociceptive effects of stressors are influenced by alterations in motivation. It is certainly conceivable, however, that the reduced responsiveness in analgesia tests is influenced by factors other than altered sensitivity to aversive stimulation.

SUMMARY

Several behavioural and neurochemical changes follow exposure to aversive stimulation and may be associated with adaptation to it, i.e. they may mediate appropriate defensive postures or oppose potential health risks (see Sklar and Anisman, 1981). It seems that numerous endogenous and exogenous factors determine the nature and magnitude of the neurochemical alterations. One of these appears to be the organism's ability to contend with the stressor by behavioural means. Thus, exposure to uncontrollable stressors reduced noradrenaline in several brain regions but escapable shock did not. In addition, behavioural coping may also influence dopamine, acetylcholine, and opioid peptide functioning.

The initial increase of neurotransmitter activity during stress may be essential for adaptation. Also sensitization or conditioning of neurochemical responses to stressors may assist adaptation on re-exposure. The reduction of transmitter levels with sufficiently severe uncontrollable stress could indicate the limits of adaptability though it is not inconceivable that the depletion itself has adaptive value. On continued exposure to aversive stimulation, increased activity of enzymes of amine synthesis restores pre-stress amine levels. Finally, subsensitivity of noradrenaline β-receptors on chronic stress application may be a compensatory response to the sustained increase of noradrenaline turnover.

Like the neurochemical consequences of stress, its behavioural consequences may depend on its controllability. These behavioural effects include escape behaviour, anti-nociception and responding to obtain electrical brain stimulation. There are indications that depression (Anisman and Zacharko, 1982) and immune functioning (e.g. Sklar and Anisman, 1979; Visintainer *et al.*, 1982) may also be influenced. That so wide a range of behavioural and psychological pathologies may be induced by aversive stimulation is not particularly surprising given the wide array of its neurochemical and hormonal consequences. However, these effects are not necessarily mediated by common mechanisms. Of course, complex behavioural effects could well reflect the interplay of different behavioural and neurochemical consequences of stress.

ACKNOWLEDGEMENT

Supported by Grant MT-6486 from the Medical Research Council of Canada and Grants A9845 and U0058 from the Natural Sciences and Engineering Research Council of Canada.

REFERENCES

Akil, H., Watson, J., Patrick, R. L., and Barchas, J. D. (1978). Stress-induced increase in endogenous opiate peptides: concurrent analgesia and its partial reversal by naloxone, in *Opiates and Endogenous Opioid Peptides* (ed H. W. Kosterlitz), pp. 63–70, Elsevier, North Holland.

Anisman, H. (1978). Neurochemical changes elicited by stress: behavioral correlates, in *Psychopharmacology of Aversively Motivated Behavior* (eds H. Anisman and G. Bignami), pp. 119–172, Plenum Press, New York.

Anisman, H. and Sklar, L. S. (1979). Catecholamine depletion upon reexposure to stress: mediation of the escape deficits produced by inescapable shock. *J. Comp. Physiol. Psychol.,* **93**, 610–625.

Anisman, H. and Sklar, L. S. (1981). Social housing conditions influence escape deficits produced by uncontrollable stress: assessment of the contribution of norepinephrine. *Behav. Neur. Biol.,* **32**, 406–427.

Anisman, H. and Zacharko, R. M. (1982). Depression: the predisposing influence of stress. *Behav. Brain Sci.,* **5**, 89–137.

Anisman, H., deCatanzaro, D., and Remington, G. (1978). Escape performance following exposure to inescapable shock: deficits in motor response maintenance. *J. Exp. Psychol.: Anim. Behav. Proc.,* **4**, 197–218.

Anisman, H., Remington, G., and Sklar, L. S. (1979a). Effects of inescapable shock on subsequent escape performance: catecholaminergic and cholinergic mediation of response initiation and maintenance. *Psychopharmacol.,* **61**, 107–124.

Anisman, H., Grimmer, L., Irwin, J., Remington, G., and Sklar, L. S. (1979b). Escape performance after inescapable shock in selectively bred lines of mice: response maintenance and catecholamine activity. *J. Comp. Physiol. Psychol.,* **93**, 229–241.

Anisman, H., Pizzino, A., and Sklar, L. S. (1980a). Coping with stress, norepinephrine depletion and escape performance. *Brain Res.,* **191**, 583–588.

Anisman, H., Suissa, A., and Sklar, L. S. (1980b). Escape deficits induced by uncontrollable stress: Antagonism by dopamine and norephinephrine agonists. *Behav. Neur. Biol.,* **28**, 34–47.

Anisman, H., Kokkinidis, L., and Sklar, L. S. (1981a). Contribution of neurochemical change to stress-induced behavioral deficits, in *Theory in Psychopharmacology, Volume I* (ed. B. J. Cooper), Academic Press, London.

Anisman, H., Glazier, S. J., and Sklar, L. S. (1981b). Cholinergic influences on escape deficits produced by uncontrollable stress. *Psychopharmacol.,* **74**, 81–87.

Anisman, H., Kokkinidis, L., and Sklar, L. S. (1982). Neurochemical consequences of stress: Contributions of adaptive processes, in *Physiological and Psychological Interactions in Response to Stress* (ed. S. Burchfield), Hemisphere, New York.

Arbuthnott, G. W. (1980). The dopamine synapse and the notion of 'pleasure centres' in the brain. *Trends in Neurosci.,* **3**, 199–200.

Ashe, V. M. and McCain, G. (1972). Comparison of one-way and shuttle-avoidance performance of gerbils and rats. *J. Comp. Physiol. Psychol.,* **80**, 293–296.

Baizman, E. R., Cox, B. M., Osman, O. H., and Goldstein, A. (1979). Experimental alterations of endorphin levels in rat pituitary. *Neuroendocrinol.,* **28**, 402–424.

Barta, A. and Yashpal, K. (1981). Regional redistribution of β-endorphin in the rat brain: the effect of stress. *Prog. Neuro-Psychopharmacol.,* **5**, 595–598.

Bignami, G. and Michalek, H. (1978). Cholinergic mechanisms in aversively motivated behavior, in *Psychopharmacology of Aversively Motivated Behavior* (eds H. Anisman and G. Bignami), Plenum Press, New York.

Blanc, G., Hervé, D., Simon, H., Lisoprawski, A., Glowinski, J., and Tassin, J. P.

(1980). Response to stress of mesocortico-frontal dopaminergic neurones in rats after long-term isolation. *Nature,* **284**, 265–267.

Blasig, J., Hollt, V., Baverle, U., and Herz, A. (1978). Involvement of endorphin in emotional hyperthermia of rats. *Life Sci.,* **23**, 2525–2532.

Bolles, R. C. (1970). Species-specific defense reactions and avoidance learning. *Psychol. Rev.,* **77**, 32–48.

Bowers, W. J., Beauchamp, C., Irwin, P. J., Zacharko, R. M., and Anisman, H. (1982). Behavioral and neurochemical consequences of acute and chronic stress. Paper presented at the 43rd Annual Meeting of the Canadian Psychological Association, Montreal.

Bruto, V. and Anisman, H. (1981). Short- and long-term effects of uncontrollable stress on exploratory patterns. *Soc. Neurosci. Abst.,* **7**, 156.

Burns, P. K., Sands, M. P., Cherek, D. R., Smith, J. E., and Lane, J. D. (1981). Monoamine changes following conditioned emotional response. *Soc. Neurosci. Abst.,* **7**, 155.

Cassens, G., Roffman, M., Kuruc, A., Orsulak, P. J., and Schildkraut, J. J. (1980). Alterations in brain norepinephrine metabolism induced by environmental stimuli previously paired with inescapable shock. *Science,* **209**, 1138–1140.

Chance, W. T., White, A. C., Krynock, G. M., and Rosecrans, J. A. (1978). Conditional fear-induced antinociception and decreased binding of (3H) N-leu-enkephalin to rat brain. *Brain Res.,* **141**, 371–374.

Cherek, D. R., Lane, J. D., Freeman, M. E., and Smith, J. E. (1980). Receptor changes following shock avoidance. *Soc. Neurosci. Abst.,* **6**, 543.

Corradini, A., Tombaugh, T. N., Zacharko, R. M., and Anisman, H. (1982). Discriminated avoidance and escape performance after pimozide treatment. Paper presented at the 43rd Annual Meeting of the Canadian Psychological Association, Montreal.

Costa, E., Tagliamonte, A., Brunello, N., and Cheney, D. L. (1980). Effect of stress on the metabolism of acetylcholine in the cholinergic pathways of extrapyramidal and limbic systems, in *Catecholamines and Stress: Recent Advances* (eds E. Usdin, R. Kvetnansky and I. J. Kopin), pp. 59–68, Elsevier, New York.

Culman, J., Kvetnansky, R., Kiss, A., Mezey, E., and Murgas, K. (1980). Interaction of serotonin and catecholamines in individual brain nuclei in adrenocortical activity regulation during stress, in *Catecholamines and Stress: Recent Advances* (eds E. Usdin, R. Kvetnansky and I. J. Kopin), pp. 69–74, Elsevier, New York.

DeVries, G. H., Chance, W. T., Payne, W. R., and Rosecrans, J. A. (1979). Effect of autoanalgesia on CNS enkephalin receptors. *Pharm. Biochem. Behav.,* **11**, 741–744.

Drugan, R. C., Grau, J. W., Maier, S. F., Madden, J., and Barchas, J. D. (1981). Cross-tolerance between morphine and the long-term analgesic reaction to inescapable shock. *Pharm. Biochem. Behav.,* **14**, 677–682.

Fadda, F., Argiolas, A., Melis, M. R., Tissari, A. H., Onali, P. L., and Gessa, G. L. (1978). Stress-induced increase in 3,4-dihydroxyphenylacetic acid (DOPAC) levels in the cerebral cortex and in nucleus accumbens: Reversal by diazepam. *Life Sci.,* **23**, 2219–2224.

Fekete, M. I. K., Szentendrei, T., Kanyicska, B., and Palkovits, M. (1981). Effects of anxiolytic drugs on the catecholamine and DOPAC (3,4-dihydroxyphenylacetic acid) levels in brain cortical areas and on corticosterone and prolactin secretion in rats subjected to stress. *Psychoneuroendocrinology,* **6**, 113–120.

German, D. C. and Bowden, D. M. (1974). Catecholamine systems as the neural substrate for intracranial self-stimulation: an hypothesis. *Brain Res.,* **73**, 381–419.

Glazer, H. I. and Weiss, J. M. (1976). Long-term interference effect: an alternative to "Learned Helplessness". *J. Exp. Psychol.: Anim. Behav. Proc.,* **2**, 202–213.

Grau, J. W., Hyson, R. L., Maier, S. F., Madden, J., and Barchas, J. D. (1981). Long-term stress-induced analgesia and activation of the opiate system. *Science,* **213**, 1409–1411.

Grossen, N. E. and Kelley, M. J. (1972). Species-specific behavior and acquisition of avoidance behavior in rats. *J. Comp. Physiol. Psychol.,* **81**, 307–310.

Guillemin, R., Vargo, T. M., Rossier, J., Minick, S., Ling, N., Rivier, C., Vale, W., and Bloom, F. (1977). β-Endorphin and adrenocorticotrophin are secreted concomitantly by the pituitary gland. *Science,* **197**, 1367–1369.

Herman, J. P., Guillonneau, D., Dantzer, R., Mormède, P., Simon, H., and LeMoal, M. (1981). Differential activation of limbic and cortical dopaminergic systems to stress and anticipation of stress. *Soc. Neurosci. Abst.,* **1**, 155.

Hingtgen, J. N., Smith, J. S., Shea, P. A., Aprison, M. H., and Gaff, T. M. (1976). Cholinergic changes during conditioned suppression in rats. *Science,* **193**, 332–334.

Iimori, K., Tanaka, M., Kohno, Y., Ida, Y., Nakagawa, R., Hoaki, Y., Tsuda, A., and Nagasaki, N. (1982). Psychological stress enhances noradrenaline turnover in specific brain regions in rats. *Pharm. Biochem. Behav.,* **16**, 637–640.

Irwin, J., Suissa, A., and Anisman, H. (1980). Differential effects of inescapable shock on escape performance and discrimination learning in a water escape task. *J. Exp. Psychol.: Anim. Behav. Proc.,* **6**, 21–40.

Irwin, J., Bowers, W., Zacharko, R. M., and Anisman, H. (1982). Stress-induced alterations of norepinephrine: cross-stressor sensitization. *Soc. Neurosci. Abstr.,* **8**, 359.

Jackson, R. L., Maier, S. F., and Coon, D. J. (1979). Long-term analgesic effects of inescapable shock and learned helplessness. *Science,* **206**, 91–93.

Jackson, R. L., Alexander, R. H., and Maier, S. F. (1980). Learned helplessness and associative deficits: effects of inescapable shock on response choice escape learning, *J. Exp. Physycol.: Anim. Behav. Proc.*, **6**, 1–20.

Karczmar, A. G., Scudder, C. L., and Richardson, D. (1973). Interdisciplinary approach to the study of behavior in related mice types, in *Neurosciences Research* (ed. I. Kopin), pp. 159–244, Academic Press, New York.

Korf, J., Aghajanian, G. K., and Roth, R. H. (1973). Increased turnover of norepinephrine in the rat cerebral cortex during stress: role of the locus coeruleus. *Neuropharmacol.,* **12**, 933–938.

Kobayashi, R. M., Palkovits, M., Kizer, J. S., Jacobowitz, D. M., and Kopin, I. J. (1976). Selective alterations of catecholamines and tyrosine hydroxylase activity in the hypothalamus following acute and chronic stress, in *Catecholamines and Stress* (eds E. Usdin, R. Kvetnansky and I. J. Kopin), pp. 29–38, Pergamon Press, Oxford.

Krieger, D. T., Liotta, A. S., Hauser, H., and Brownstein, M. J. (1979). Effect of stress, adrenocorticotropin or corticosteroid treatment, adrenalectomy or hypophysectomy on hypothalamic immunoreactive adrenocorticotropin concentrations. *Endocrinol.,* **105**, 737–742.

Kvetnansky, R., Mitro, A., Palkovits, M., Brownstein, M., Torda, T., Vigas, M., and Mikulaj, L. (1976). Catecholamines in individual hypothalamic nuclei in stressed rats, in *Catecholamines and Stress* (eds E. Usdin, R. Kvetnansky and I. J. Kopin), pp. 39–50, Pergamon Press, Oxford.

Kvetnansky, R., Palkovits, M., Mitro, A., Torda, T., and Mikulaj, L. (1977). Catecholamines in individual hypothalamic nuclei of acutely and repeatedly stressed rats. *Neuroendocrin.,* **23**, 257–267.

Lewis, J. W., Cannon, J. T., and Liebeskind, J. C. (1980). Opioid and nonopioid mechanisms of stress analgesia. *Science,* **208**, 623–625.

Lewis, J. W., Sherman, J. E., and Liebeskind, J. C. (1981). Opioid and nonopioid stress and analgesia: assessment of tolerance and cross-tolerance with morphine. *J. Neurosci.,* **1**, 358–363.

Madden, J. N., Akil, H., Patrick, R. L., and Barchas, J. D. (1977). Stress-induced parallel changes in central opioid levels and pain responsiveness in the rat. *Nature,* **265**, 358–360.

Mah, C., Suissa, A., and Anisman, H. (1980). Dissociation of antinociception and escape deficits induced by stress in mice. *J. Comp. Physiol. Psychol.,* **94**, 1160–1171.

Maier, S. F. and Testa, T. J. (1975). Failure to learn escape by rats previously exposed to inescapable shock is partly produced by associative interference. *J. Comp. Physiol. Psychol.,* **88**, 554.

Maier, S. F. and Seligman, M. E. P. (1976). Learned helplessness: theory and evidence. *J. Exp. Psychol.: Gen.,* **105**, 3–46.

Maier, S. F. and Jackson, R. L. (1979). Learned helplessness: all of us were right (and wrong): inescapable shock has multiple effects, in *The Psychology of Learning and Motivation, Vol. 13* (ed. G. Bower), Academic Press, New York.

Maier, S. F., Albin, R. W., and Testa, T. J. (1973). Failure to learn to escape in rats previously exposed to inescapable shock depends on nature of escape response. *J. Comp. Physiol. Psychol.,* **85**, 581–592.

Maier, S. F., Davies, S., Grau, J. W., Jackson, R. L., Morrison, D. H., Moye, T., Madden, J., and Barchas, J. D. (1980). Opiate antagonists and the long-term analgesia reaction induced by inescapable shock in rats. *J. Comp. Physiol. Psychol.,* **94**, 1172–1183.

Maier, S. F., Drugan, R. C., and Grau, J. W. (1982). Controllability, coping behavior and stress-induced analgesia in the rat. *Pain,* **12**, 47–56.

Modigh, K. (1976). Influence of social stress on brain catecholamine mechanisms, in *Catecholamines and Stress* (eds E. Usdin, R. Kvetnansky and I. J. Kopin), pp. 17–28, Pergamon Press, Oxford.

Moye, T. B., Coon, D. J., Grau, J. W., and Maier, S. F. (1981). Therapy and immunization of long-term analgesia in rats. *Learn. Motiv.,* **12**, 133–148.

Nakagawa, R., Tanaka, M., Kohno, Y., Noda, Y., and Nagasaki, N. (1981). Regional responses of rat brain noradrenergic neurons to acute intense stress. *Pharm. Biochem. Behav.,* **14**, 729–732.

Nomura, S., Watanabe, M., Ukei, N., and Nakazawa, T. (1981). Stress and β-adrenergic receptor binding in the rat's brain. *Brain Res.,* **224**, 199.

Palkovits, M., Brownstein, M., Kizer, J. S., Saavedra, J. M. and Kopin, I. J. (1976). Effect of stress on serotonin and tryptophan hydroxylase activity of brain nuclei, in *Catecholamines and Stress* (eds. E. Usdin, R. Kvetnansky and I. J. Kopin), Pergamon Press, New York.

Petty, F. and Sherman, A. (1982). A neurochemical differentiation between exposure to stress and the development of learned helplessness. *Drug Devel. Res.,* **2**, 43–45.

Ritter, S. and Pelzer, N. L. (1978). Magnitude of stress-induced brain norepinephrine depletion varies with age. *Brain Res.,* **152**, 170–175.

Rossier, J., Guillemin, R., and Bloom, F. (1978). Foot-shock induced stress decreases Leu^5-enkephalin immunoreactivity in rat hypothalamus. *Eur. J. Pharmacol.,* **48**, 465–466.

Saavedra, J. M. (1980). Brain and pineal adrenaline: its level, synthesis and possible function in stress, in *Stress and Catecholamines: Recent Advances* (eds E. Usdin, R. Kvetnansky and I. J. Kopin), pp. 37–46, Elsevier, New York.

Saavedra, J. M., Kvetnansky, R., and Kopin, I. J. (1979). Adrenaline, noradrenaline and dopamine levels in specific brainstem areas of acutely immobilized rats. *Brain Res.,* **160**, 271–280.

Santagostino, A., Cocchi, D., Giagnoni, E., Gori, E., Muller, E., and Ferri, S. (1978). Some relationships between endorphins and pituitary hormones, in *Advances in Biochemical Pharmacology, Vol. 18* (eds. E. Costa and M. Trabucchi), pp. 175–181, Raven Press, New York.

Sherman, A. D. and Petty, F. (1980). Neurochemical basis of the action of anti-depressants on learned helplessness. *Behav. Neur. Biol.,* **30**, 119–134.

Shettleworth, S. J. (1972). Constraints on learning, in *Advances in the Study of Behavior. Vol. 4* (eds D. S. Lehrmann, R. A. Hinde and E. Shaw), Academic Press, New York.

Sklar, L. S. and Anisman, H. (1979). Stress and coping factors influence tumor growth. *Science,* **205**, 513–515.

Sklar, L. S., and Anisman, H. (1981). Contributions of stress and coping to cancer development and growth, in *Stress and Cancer* (eds K. Bammer and B. H. Newberry), pp. 98–136, C. J. Hogrefe, Toronto.

Stolk, J. M., Conner, R. L., Levine, S., and Barchas, J. D. (1974). Brain norepinephrine metabolism and shock induced fighting behavior in rats: differential effects of shock and fighting on the neurochemical response to a common footshock stimulus. *J. Pharm. Exp. Ther.,* **190**, 193–209.

Stone, E. A. (1975). Stress and catecholamines, in *Catecholamines and Behavior Volume II* (ed A. J. Friedhoff), Plenum Press, New York.

Stone, E. A. (1979). Reduction by stress of norepinephrine-stimulated accumulation of cyclic AMP in rat cerebral cortex. *J. Neurochem.,* **32**, 1335–1337.

Stone, E. A. (1980). Subsensitivity to norepinephrine as a link between adaptation to stress and antidepressant therapy: an Hypothesis. *Res. Comm. Psychol. Psychiat. Behav.,* **4**, 241–255.

Telner, J. I. and Singhal, R. L. (1981). Effects of nortriptyline treatment on learned helplessness in the rat. *Pharm. Biochem. Behav.,* **14**, 823.

Testa, T. J. (1974). Causal relationships and the acquisition of avoidance responses. *Psychol. Rev.,* **81**, 491–505.

Thierry, A. M. (1973). Effects of stress on the metabolism of serotonin and norepinephrine in the central nervous system of the rat, in *Hormones, Metabolism and Stress: Recent Progress and Perspectives* (ed S. Nemeth), Publishing House of the Slovak Academy of Science, Bratislava.

Thierry, A. M., Javoy, F., Glowinski, J., and Kety, S. S. (1968). Effects of stress on the metabolism of norepinephrine, dopamine and serotonin in the central nervous system of the rat. *J. Pharm. Exp. Ther.,* **163**, 163–171.

Thierry, A. M., Blanc, G., and Glowinski, J. (1971). Effect of stress on the disposition of catecholamines localized in various intraneuronal storage forms in the brainstem of the rat. *J. Neurochem.,* **18**, 449–461.

Thierry, A. M., Tassin, J. P., Blanc, G., and Glowinski, J. (1976). Selective activation of the mesocortical DA system by stress. *Nature,* **263**, 242–244.

Tissari, A. H., Argiolas, A., Fadda, F., Serra, G., and Gessa, L. (1979). Footshock stress accelerates non-striatal dopamine synthesis without activating tyrosine hydroxylase. *Arch. Pharmacol.,* **308**, 155–158.

Usdin, E., Kvetnansky, R., and Kopin, I. J. (1976). *Stress and Catecholamines*, Pergamon Press, Oxford.

Usdin, E., Kvetnansky, R., and Kopin, I. J. (1980). *Catecholamines and Stress: Recent Advances*, Elsevier, New York.

Versteeg, D. H. G., DeKloet, E. R., and DeWied, D. (1978). Interaction of endorphins with brain catecholamine systems, in *Characteristics and Function of Opioids* (eds Van Ree and Terenius), pp. 323–331, Elsevier, North-Holland.

Visintainer, M. A., Volpicelli, J. R., and Seligman, M. E. P. (1982). Tumor rejection in rats after inescapable shock. *Science,* **216**, 437–439.

Wahlsten, D. (1980). A critique of the concept of heritability and heredity in behavioral genetics, in *Theoretical Advances in Behavior Genetics* (eds J. R. Royce and L. P. Mos), Sijthoff and Noordhoff, Germantown.

Watson, S. J., Akil, H., Richard, C. W., and Barchas, J. D. (1978). Evidence for two separate opiate peptide neuronal systems. *Nature,* **275**, 226–228.

Weber, E., Voigt, K. H., and Martin, R. (1978). Concomitant storage of ACTH and endorphin-like immunoreactivity in secretory granules of anterior pituitary corticotrophs. *Brain Res.,* **157**, 385–390.

Weiss, J. M., Glazer, H. I., Pohorecky, L. A. (1976). Coping behavior and neurochemical changes: An alternative explanation for the original "learned helplessness" experiments, in *Animal Models in Human Psychobiology* (eds G. Serban and A. Kling), Plenum Press, 1976.

Weiss, J. M., Glazer, H. I., Pohorecky, L. A., Bailey, W. H., and Schneider, L. H. (1979). Coping behavior and stress-induced behavioral depression: studies of the role of brain catecholamines, in *The Psychobiology of the Depressive Disorders* (ed R. A. Depue), Academic Press, New York.

Weiss, J M. Goodman, P. A., Losito, B. G., Corrigan, S., Charry, J. M., and Bailey, W. H. (1981). Behavioral depression produced by an uncontrollable stressor: relationship to norepinephrine, dopamine and serotonin levels in various regions of rat brain, *Brain Res. Rev.*, **3**, 167–205.

Welch, A. S. and Welch, B. L. (1968). Reduction of norepinephrine in the lower brainstem by psychological stimulus. *Proc. Natl Acad. Sci.,* **60**, 478–481.

Welch, B. L. and Welch, A. S. (1970). Control of brain catecholamines and serotonin during acute stress and after d-amphetamine by natural inhibition of monoamine oxidase: an hypothesis, in *Amphetamines and Related Compounds* (eds E. Costa and S. Garattini), pp. 415–445, Raven Press, New York.

Wimer, R. E., Norman, R., and Eleftheriou, B. E. (1973). Serotonin levels in hippocampus: striking variations associated with mouse strain and treatment. *Brain Res.,* **63**, 397–401.

Wise, R. A. (1978). Catecholamine theories of reward: a critical review. *Brain Res.,* **152**, 215–248.

Wise, R. A. (1980). 'Yes, but!...' a response to Arbuthnott from Roy Wise, *Trends Neurosci.,* **3**, 200.

Zacharko, R. M., Bowers, W. J., Kokkinidis, L., and Anisman, H. (1982). Alteration of intracranial self-stimulation in mice following inescapable stress. *Soc. Neurosci. Abst.* **8**, 898.

Zajaczkowska, M. N. (1975). Acetylcholine content in the central and peripheral nervous system and its synthesis in the rat brain during stress and post-stress exhaustion. *Acta Physiol. Pol.,* **26**, 493–497.

Stress-induced Analgesia
Edited by M. D. Tricklebank and G. Curzon

CHAPTER 4

Physiological approaches to counter-irritation phenomena

D. LE BARS, B. CALVINO, L. VILLANUEVA, and S. CADDEN

Counter-irritation phenomena, i.e. the paradoxical pain relieving effects of pain elicited from heterotopic body areas, have been known for centuries. In fact, most popular methods of practising medicine include the therapeutic use of counter-irritation and it has been subjected to repeated rediscovery by scientists. However, the older literature devoted to this subject is not always easy to interpret, due to various aspects of medical practice prior to the discovery and use of major analgesics (e.g. claims of efficacy of treatment can imply either recovery or only pain relief) and also due to lack of data on the psychological profiles of suffering patients (e.g., see Sternbach, 1976). Further difficulties in this field arise from what we know today about the complex integrative processes associated with pain sensation, and in particular the multiple interactions between peripheral inputs as early as the first relays in the central nervous system. However, two decades of electrophysiological and clinical investigations have led to some conclusions which allow attempts at re-interpreting older observations, but, as will be seen, these attempts need to take account of numerous factors.

In the present chapter we will briefly summarize work on counter-irritation phenomena and their possible underlying neurophysiological mechanisms. The eventual involvement of such mechanisms in some forms of 'stress induced analgesia' will also be considered.

I THE COUNTER-IRRITATION PHENOMENA

A Clinical approaches

As mentioned above, counter-irritation phenomena have been known since antiquity. They have often been used in treatments of inflammatory processes, for example in 'cupping'. The application of most counter-irritants produced more or less bearable pain as a treatment of pain of pathological origin. One of the best examples is probably the use of the discharge of electric eel, as a pain-reliever. As recently reviewed by Kane and Taub (1975), the Greeks and probably the Egyptians knew about these effects which are referred to in numerous manuscripts. Various non-Western (e.g. Chinese) medical procedures also included (and still include) counter-irritation as a pain-relieving technique.

In 1956, Wand-Tetley reviewed a series of old counter-irritation methods used for treatment of rheumatic diseases. Most of them were undoubtedly painful: for instance, 'cupping' when associated with scarification of the skin, cautery, moxibustion or blisters. A passage from his article is reproduced below.

> Blisters had a multitude of uses. They could be applied almost anywhere on the body, but the commonest sites appear to have been the scalp, behind the ears, the neck, and the soles of the feet. Ordinary rubefacients of the nineteenth century were mustard, ammonia, camphor, oil of turpentine, and the dilute mineral acids; and the usual blistering agents (or vesicatories, as they were called) were ointment of tartar emetic, silver nitrate, and cantharides powder. But for blistering, as Syme (1863) tells us, "when the effect is wished to be strong and immediate, recourse may be had to boiling water, or the concentrated mineral acids".
>
> Once a blister had been raised, it was either punctured to release its fluid, or (when the blister was to be kept open) the detached skin was removed and the raw surface dressed in a particular manner. Syme says: "In order to prolong the irritation of blisters, it used to be customary to dress the raw part with an ointment containing savine leaves, or the powder of cantharides, which prevented it from healing, and maintained a discharge of matter".

Distinction between the direct hypoalgesic and anti-inflammatory purposes of such treatments are not clear. However, 'strong and immediate effects' most probably refer to analgesia.

Such clinical practices progressively disappeared in modern occidental medicine when analgesic and anti-inflammatory drugs became available. It should be stressed however that country people still use this principle when they squeeze the muzzle ('twitch') of a bull-calf during castration in the absence of any medication. The use of moxibustion in Chinese popular veterinary medicine is illustrated in Figure 4.1.

The use of electrical stimulation was introduced in the nineteenth century as a pain-relieving method and, although a subject of controversy it has commonly been used in Western medicine (see references in Kane and Taub, 1975). In the light of recent neurophysiological knowledge (see below), it appears that several mechanisms might have been brought into play by such

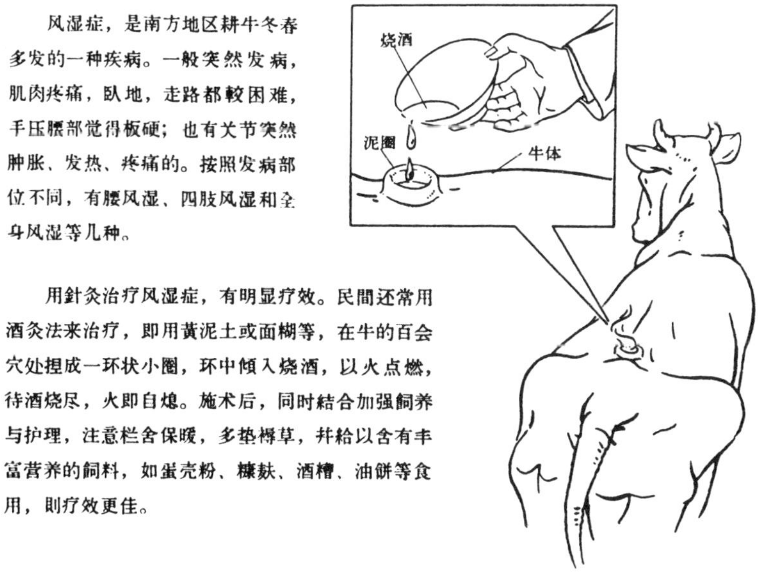

Figure 4.1 Example of the hypoalgesic effect of moxibustion as used in Chinese traditional veterinary practice (from a veterinary acupuncture plate sold in Peking in 1971).

Translation. In the south of China, draught cattle often exhibit rheumatic diseases in winter and spring. The symptoms appear suddenly with myalgia associated with lumbar stiffness and laborious walk. Lumbar, limb or generalized rheumatisms are observed.

Acupuncture is strongly effective against rheumatic syndromes. Popular treatment often uses moxibustion with alcohol: first one has to make a kind of ring using clay set on the lumbar 'Bai-Hui' point of the diseased cow; then alcohol is poured into it which must be consumed until extinction … .

Note in this text the implicit relevance of acupuncture to the counter-irritation effects of an intense burn.

techniques, depending on the nature of the current used and/or the part of the body to which it was applied. In some cases, segmental inhibitory mechanisms induced by low intensity currents (see Section II A) were most probably the underlying mechanisms. In others, the practices clearly involved counter-irritation phenomena. (i.e., Sarlandière, 1825; Trousseau and Pidoux, 1851; Duchenne de Boulogne, 1855). In the English translation from the French edition of his textbook (1869), De Niemeyer refers to the treatment of neuralgia:

> The application of electricity must be counted as being amongst the best means of fulfilling these conditions. The best results are often obtained by induced current as well as by constant current. […].

> The application of induced current in the fashion which we are going to describe, is very painful; it is only when the sick are certain of favourable results through their own experience, that they agree to submit themselves to the treatment patiently, albeit normally, with sighs and moans as signs of their suffering. At the point where the current has acted on the skin, an erythema with an adequately long duration, occurs. [...].
>
> A means which is put to use in the neuralgias, very much more than the use of induced current, is the use of constant current. [...]. The application of constant current does not initially produce as strong a pain, but it soon expands into a disagreeable sensation of burning and tingling, which increases progressively and becomes exacerbated to an intolerable degree if a large number of elements are used. The modifications of the skin produced by the constant current at its site of application are much stronger, if the electrodes are kept in place for a given time, than those seen with the induced current. They not only consist of a strong erythema, as considerable swelling of the skin and an increase in the volume of subcutaneous areas, but in addition, especially at the point of application of the positive pole, weals and patches of rash develop, the surface of which is covered with a slough if the electricity acts for a longer or shorter time.

More recently, painful electrical stimulation of the skin was reintroduced in the treatment of chronic pain (Melzack, 1975; Jeans, 1979) and described as 'hypoalgesia by hyperstimulation'. Interestingly, the hypoalgesia induced by some forms of acupuncture or electroacupuncture has been postulated as being related to counter-irritation phenomena (Wand-Tetley, 1956; Fox and Melzack, 1976a, 1976b; Levine *et al.*, 1976; Melzack *et al.*, 1977). Based on a wide clinical experience, the conclusion reached by Mann (1974) was that acupuncture stimulation must be both as painful and as strong as the patient will tolerate for a reliable pain-relieving effect to occur.

Finally, intense cold ('ice massage') applied to the hand has been reported to relieve dental pain (Melzack *et al.*, 1980a) and related methods have been used for the treatment of muscular (Grant, 1964; Mennell, 1975) and low-back pain (Melzack *et al.*, 1980b).

Further clinical evidence for the existence of a diffuse pain inhibitory system triggered by pain of peripheral origin is the observation that organic pain raises pain thresholds in other areas of the body (Hazouri and Mueller, 1950; Merskey and Evans, 1975).

B Experimental approaches in man

To our knowledge, the first experimental investigation of counterirritation phenomena was made by Duncker (1937). Referring to the practices we have mentioned above, he noted that

> in the olden days where modern anaesthetics were not yet discovered it was one of the functions of the dentist's assistant to pinch the patient at the critical moment,

and he undertook 'experiments on the mutual influence of pains' induced mechanically on right and left forearms respectively. He concluded that in about 40 cases and without exception, a pain A (*active*) induced a decrease of a distant and simultaneous pain P (*passive*) if A was stronger than P and, if so, in proportion to A's relative intensity. Further experiments allowed him to conclude

> 'I never encountered any chance evidence that quality of A or distance between A and P were playing a part. Pain in a toe caused by contact with a hot-water bottle would readily yield under the influence of pain inflicted by pinching the lobe of an ear'.

Hardy *et al.* (1940) also reached similar conclusions. One of their experiments is illustrated in Figure 4.2: the pain threshold was measured using radiant heat application to the forehead; a sphygmomanometer cuff placed around the left arm was then inflated to a pressure of 200 mm Hg which resulted in a progressive pain sensation associated with a disappearance of other sensations emanating from this arm. The threshold for pain elicited by means of thermal radiation of the forehead increased in a strikingly parallel fashion to the pain sensation elicited from the arm. Further investigations by the same group (Berlin *et al.*, 1958), using two radiant heat dolorimeters applied to various body areas confirmed these results and allowed them to state that both pain and reflex threshold were affected by what they called 'extinction of pain'.

Gammon and Starr (1941), using several types of counter-irritant (cold, heat, mechanical, electrical), described a similar phenomenon, the most effective method being the application of painful cold (4–10 °C). They mainly investigated the effects of counter-irritants applied over the painful area (i.e., near the body surface where the conditioned painful stimulus was applied) but noticed that counter-irritation applied elsewhere was 'by no means ineffectual'. Similarly, Parsons and Goetzl (1945) reported that painful cold applied to a leg was able to increase the dental pain threshold measured by using electrical stimulation of a tooth.

In a recent study, we undertook a psychophysiological and electrophysiological study of counter-irritation (Le Bars *et al.*, 1983). The experimental procedure (Figure 4.3A) consisted of stimulating the right sural nerve and studying the variations in the resultant thresholds for pain and the nociceptive flexor reflex RIII (see Willer, 1977) during the application of various painful stimuli to the left hand or nose. It was found that muscular pain (induced by

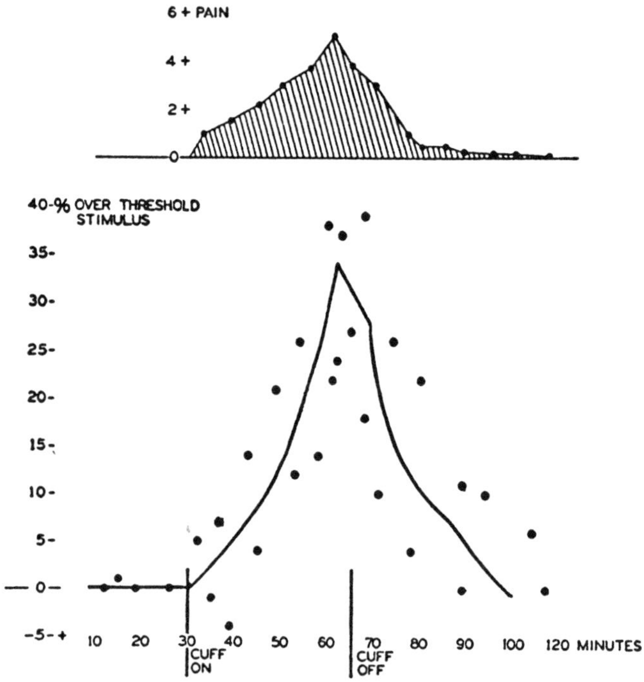

FIGURE 4.2 The effect of arresting the blood flow to the left arm upon the pain threshold on the forehead in man (from Hardy *et al.*, 1940).

The upper shaded area represents the subjective estimates of the pain caused by the ischaemia in the arm (induced by a sphygmomanometer cuff wound above the elbow and inflated to a pressure of 200 mmHg).

The pain threshold was estimated by applying thermal radiation to the forehead (lower curve). Note the parallelism between the pain sensation arising from the arm and the increase in pain threshold on the forehead.

muscular contraction during ischaemia), pressure pain, cold pain (6 °C) or heat pain, all increased the thresholds for both pain and the RIII reflex in the right leg. Figure 4.3B illustrates results obtained with heat counter-irritation. Note that using an heterotopic thermal stimulus, the threshold for obtaining inhibition of the spinal nociceptive reflex and a corresponding decrease in pain sensation ranged from 44 to 45 °C, and that these inhibitory effects then increased as a function of the temperature.

These results strongly suggest that the effects are triggered once the peripheral stimulus reaches an intensity which can produce a painful sensation. Indeed, the threshold for pain sensation induced by heating the skin is approximately 45 °C

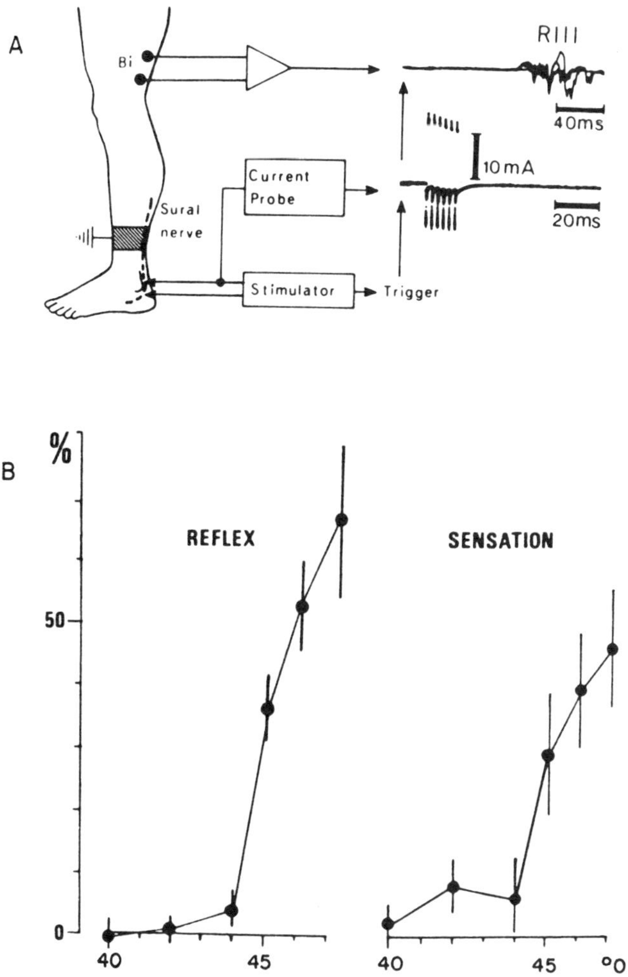

FIGURE 4.3 Effects of heterotopic thermal stimuli on a nociceptive flexion reflex and the related pain sensation in man (Le Bars *et al.*, 1983).

A — Experimental design: the right sural nerve is stimulated percutaneously at the ankle and the nociceptive reflex response (RIII) is recorded from the biceps femoris muscle. The threshold for obtaining such a reflex is well correlated with the threshold for pain sensation (Willer, 1977). Both these electrophysiological and psychophysiological responses (the latter being estimated on an arbitrary scale) are provoked by the immersion of the contralateral (left) hand in a stirred water bath maintained at various temperatures.

B — Results: effects of the application of various temperatures on the hand on the RIII reflex threshold (left) and the pain threshold (right) induced by sural nerve stimulation Note that both thresholds were increased in a parallel fashion when the provoking stimulus reached a noxious level (>45°C).

(Hardy *et al.*, 1951) and a linear dolorimetric scale is perceived in the 44–50 °C range (Adair *et al.*, 1968; Lamotte and Campbell, 1978).

C Behavioural approaches in animals

The experimental approach to the study of counter-irritation phenomena in animals is not easy for several reasons. Apart from the general difficulties of studying pain in animals there are problems related to the necessary application of two noxious stimuli — one 'active' and affecting the response to the latter 'passive' stimulus. Results may be influenced by the mutual effects of these stimuli while the 'active' stimulus might induce stress reactions other than those specifically related to nociception.

However, experimental data suggests that counter-irritation phenomena can be observed in animal models. For instance, in the cat, stimulation of tooth pulp at an obviously noxious intensity can increase the threshold for escape behaviour induced by footshock by up to 70% (Anderson *et al.*, 1976). In rodents, sustained pinch applied to the paw or tail (Colpaert *et al.*, 1978), noxious cold applied to the entire body (Bodnar *et al.*, 1982), and various electrical shocks applied to the feet or tail (Chesher and Chan, 1977; Hayes *et al.*, 1978; Buckett, 1979, 1981; Lewis *et al.*, 1980, 1981; Hutson *et al.*, 1981; Tricklebank *et al.*, 1982; Watkins *et al.*, 1982a; Watkins and Mayer, 1982b; and see refs in other contributions to this volume) can induce potent hypoalgesic effects. Visceral nociceptive stimuli can also induce hypoalgesia in behavioural testing (Hayes *et al.*, 1978; Kraus *et al.*, 1981, 1982; Chapman and Way, 1982). In a recent study, we used such a visceral stimulus to evalute the reciprocal influences of the so-called 'active' and 'passive' stimuli. The behavioural response was the vocalization produced by electrical stimulation of the tail. Intraperitoneal (i.p.) injection of acetic acid (pH 2.7) induced a rise in the threshold for vocalization (Figure 4.4A). Acetic acid can trigger behavioural responses which are often used as a model for pain in the behavioural screening of putative analgesic drugs (Niemegeers *et al.*, 1975). This is illustrated in Figure 4.4B in which i.p. administration of acetic acid resulted in long lasting writhing behaviour. However, as shown in Figure 4.4B(b), the subcutaneous insertion of needles in both sides of the rat's tail, significantly reduced this behaviour. Moreover, during testing of the threshold for vocalization induced by electrical stimulation of the tail using the two subcutaneously implanted needles (i.e., during the experiment ilustrated in Figure 4.4A), writhing behaviour in response to i.p. acetic acid disappeared almost completely (Figure 4.4B(c)). In other words, these results suggest that mutual interactions exist between the behaviours triggered from the viscerae and the tail respectively.

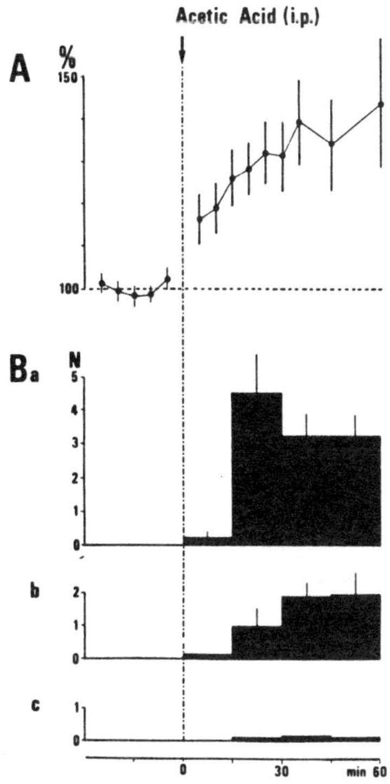

Figure 4.4 Effects of intraperitoneal administration of acetic acid (pH 2.7) in the rat (groups of 16 animals in each case).

A — The threshold for vocalization induced by electrical stimulation of the tail (50 Hz, 2 ms width, 500 ms duration). Results are expressed as a percentage of the mean of five control responses in each individual case. Note that the visceral noxious stimulus induced a rise in the threshold for vocalization.

B — Writhing behaviour (ordinate: writhings during 15 min). (a) Control animals (classical writhing test). (b) Animals having needles inserted subcutaneously on both sides of the tail. (c) Animals having needles inserted subcutaneously on both sides of the tail and tested for vocalization threshold (i.e., during experiment illustrated in A).

Note the mutual influence of the visceral and the tail nociceptive stimuli on the squeaking and writhing reactions respectively.

II POSSIBLE NEUROPHYSIOLOGICAL BASIS FOR COUNTER-IRRITATION PHENOMENA

The transmission of nociceptive messages is powerfully modulated as early as the first relays of the central nervous system, i.e. at the levels of the spinal dorsal horn or trigeminal nucleus. The 'gate-control theory' (Melzack and Wall, 1965) was an attempt to summarize schematically the data relevant to these controls, and, although its details have been subject to debate (see reference in Nathan, 1976; Wall, 1978), it is now well established that the transmission of nociceptive messages is under the influence of both segmental mechanisms and systems involving supraspinal structures (see references in Zimmermann, 1977; Fields and Basbaum, 1978; Wall, 1978; Willis and Coggeshall, 1978; Besson *et al.*, 1982). The physiological observation that somatic stimuli can trigger these controls, is most relevant to the clinical and therapeutical approaches to pain as it indicates that highly complex interactions occur before a noxious message reaches the brain. Schematically, at least two main types of system seem to be involved in these controls, depending on the innocuous or nociceptive nature of the stimulus applied.

We would like to emphasize that pure noxious stimuli are often difficult to define in experimental situations. As an illustration of this, it is clear that high intensity electrical stimulation of somatic areas activate both low and high threshold afferents resulting in an activation of several inhibitory systems. For this reason, although mainly devoted to inhibitory systems triggered by noxious inputs, this section will also briefly summarize current data relevant to inhibitory systems triggered by innocuous inputs.

A Inhibitory processes triggered by innocuous inputs

It is now well established that the electrical activation of large diameter peripheral myelinated fibres is able to inhibit the firing of dorsal horn neurones induced by noxious stimulation (Mendell, 1966; Wagman and Price, 1969; Price and Wagman, 1970; Gregor and Zimmermann, 1972; Brown *et al.*, 1973; Handwerker *et al.*, 1975; Cervero *et al.*, 1976). Such inhibitory effects are essentially metameric in nature and have been particularly studied on convergent neurones, i.e. those which respond to both innocuous and noxious stimuli applied to a well delimited area of the body (excitatory receptive field). Analogous inhibitory effects can also be induced by the stimulation of the dorsal columns (Hillman and Wall, 1969; Handwerker *et al.*, 1975; Foreman *et al.*, 1976; Lindblom *et al.*, 1977), which activate the same kind of fibres and, via antidromic processes, would probably trigger the same mechanisms. Finally the activities of a large proportion of convergent neurones can be inhibited by the application of innocuous mechanical stimuli to an area surrounding the excitatory receptive field (inhibitory receptive field) (Wall, 1967; Hillman and Wall, 1969; Wagman and Price, 1969; Besson, *et al.*, 1974).

The nature of the inhibitions observed in electrophysiological experiments has been a controversial subject. It is generally accepted today that they involve both presynaptic (Koketsu, 1956; Eccles and Krnjevic, 1959; Eccles *et al.*, 1963; Hodge, 1972; Whitehorn and Burgess, 1973) and postsynaptic (Hongo *et al.*, 1968; Price *et al.*, 1971; Zieglgänsberger and Herz, 1971; Besson *et al.*, 1974) mechanisms. Finally, neurones located within the substantia gelatinosa — SG, lamina II of Rexed (1952, 1954) — are most probably involved in at least some of these effects (see refs in Cervero and Iggo, 1980; Wall, 1980; Besson *et al.*, 1982).

These electrophysiological results could represent the neuronal basis of hypoalgesia obtained in humans by high frequency, low intensity electrical stimulation of peripheral nerves and dorsal roots (Wall and Sweet, 1967; Meyer and Fields, 1972; Satran and Goldstein, 1973; Campbell and Taub, 1973; Nathan and Wall, 1974; Long and Hagfors, 1975; Eriksson and Sjölund, 1976) or dorsal columns (Shealy *et al.*, 1970; Nashold and Friedman, 1972; Nielson *et al.*, 1975). It is important to note, however, that the time constants of these clinical and physiological phenomena are quite different as pain can be alleviated for hours in patients whereas neuronal inhibitions last, at most, for several seconds.

B Inhibitory processes triggered by noxious inputs

(a) Diffuse noxious inhibitory controls

The activity of certain dorsal horn neurones can be strongly inhibited by noxious inputs. Since such effects do not appear to be somatotopically organized but concern the entire body, they have been called diffuse noxious inhibitory controls (Le Bars *et al.*, 1979a, b). Indeed, convergent neurones, i.e. those receiving both low and high threshold afferents, whether recorded in the dorsal horn or in its homologous structure for the face, the trigeminal nucleus caudalis, are under the influence of such controls (Le Bars *et al.*, 1979a; Dickenson *et al.*, 1980a). In the anaesthetized rat the activities of almost all convergent neurones, including those projecting toward the thalamus (Dickenson and Le Bars, 1982), can be blocked by various noxious stimuli applied to parts of the body distant from the excitatory receptive fields. These inhibitory effects concern all types of neuronal activity whether spontaneous or induced by noxious or innocuous stimuli. Finally, this property appears to be specific to convergent neurones since the other neuronal types commonly encountered within the dorsal horn or the trigeminal nucleus caudalis (specifically nociceptive, non-nociceptive, cold responsive, or proprioceptive neurones) are not affected (Le Bars *et al.*, 1979b; Dickenson *et al.*, 1980a).

For example, when studying lumbar convergent neurones with peripheral receptive fields located on the ipsilateral hindpaw extremities, this type of inhibition can be triggered from widespread areas of the body, e.g. the tail, the contralateral hindpaw, the forepaws, the ears, the nose, or the viscerae. While non-noxious stimuli are totally ineffective, very strong inhibitions occur on applying mechanical, thermal, chemical, or electrical stimuli at noxious levels. Also, effects commonly persist for up to 20 min after the stimuli are withdrawn. Both the strength and long duration of these inhibitions are illustrated in Figure 4.5 in which the response of a convergent neurone to a sustained pinch of its receptive field is affected by distant thermal and mechanical noxious stimuli.

The strength of the effect is actually related to the strength of the above stimulus. For example, the threshold for triggering diffuse noxious inhibitory control by a thermal stimulus is between 40 and 44°C and a very significant correlation is observed between higher stimulus temperatures (44–52°C) and the degree of inhibition (Le Bars *et al.*, 1981a). This is illustrated in Figure 4.6; thus, the responses of the neurone to C fibre activation, induced by transcutaneous electrical stimulation of its receptive field located on the extremity of a hindpaw, are strongly depressed by the immersion of the tail in a 48°C or a 52°C water bath, whereas a slighter effect is induced at 44°C. This strongly suggests that the recruitment of peripheral nocicpetors is needed to trigger the inhibitory control. Indeed, in the monkey, polymodal C nociceptors (the most important group of nociceptors (see reference in Besson *et al.*, 1982)) increased their firing rate in relation to the temperature applied on their receptive field in the 45–50°C range. Also, in a study in man in which both psychological and electrophysiological approaches were used, Gybels *et al.* (1979) demonstrated a good correlation between the activity of polymodal nociceptors and the subject's sensation as estimated on a dolorimetric scale, during the application of thermal stimuli. These data illustrate the close correlations that exist (using thermal stimuli) between the activity of peripheral nociceptors, pain sensation and the strength of the counter-irritation phenomena in man, and also between their activity and the strength of diffuse noxious inhibitory controls in animals.

Using electrical conditioning stimuli, a similar relationship can also be observed (Figure 4.7) as increasing the current intensity towards noxious levels results in a corresponding increase of inhibitory effects.

A similar relationship can also be seen using electrical stimuli. Increasing the current intensity toward noxious levels results in a corresponding increase in inhibitory effects (Figure 4.7). The close correlation between pain reactions and the strength of diffuse noxious inhibitory controls is further suggested by our finding (Dickenson *et al.*, 1979) that the threshold intensity of shock to the

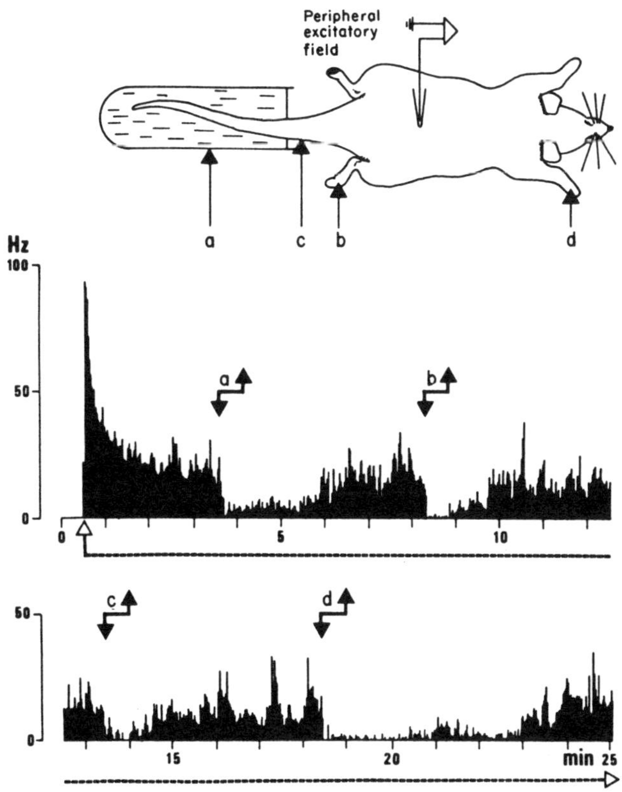

Figure 4.5 Inhibitory effects induced by various heterotopic noxious stimuli upon the response of a convergent neurone to sustained pinch (from Cadden *et al.*, 1983).

The application of sustained pinch (open arrowhead, broken line) to the peripheral excitatory field of the lumbar convergent neurone located on a hindpaw extremity resulted in a phasic response followed by a tonic discharge. Various stimuli (filled arrowheads) induced strong inhibitory effects followed by long lasting after effects. (a) immersion of the tail in a 52 °C water bath; (b) pinch of the contralateral hindpaw; (c) pinch of the tail; (d) pinch of a forepaw.

tail necessary to induce vocalization in the freely moving rat (2.14 mA) is rather similar to that necessary for the inhibition of convergent neurones (2.94 mA) (Le Bars *et al.*, 1979a).

(b) Propriospinal mechanisms

It is important to note that in addition to diffuse noxious inhibitory control,

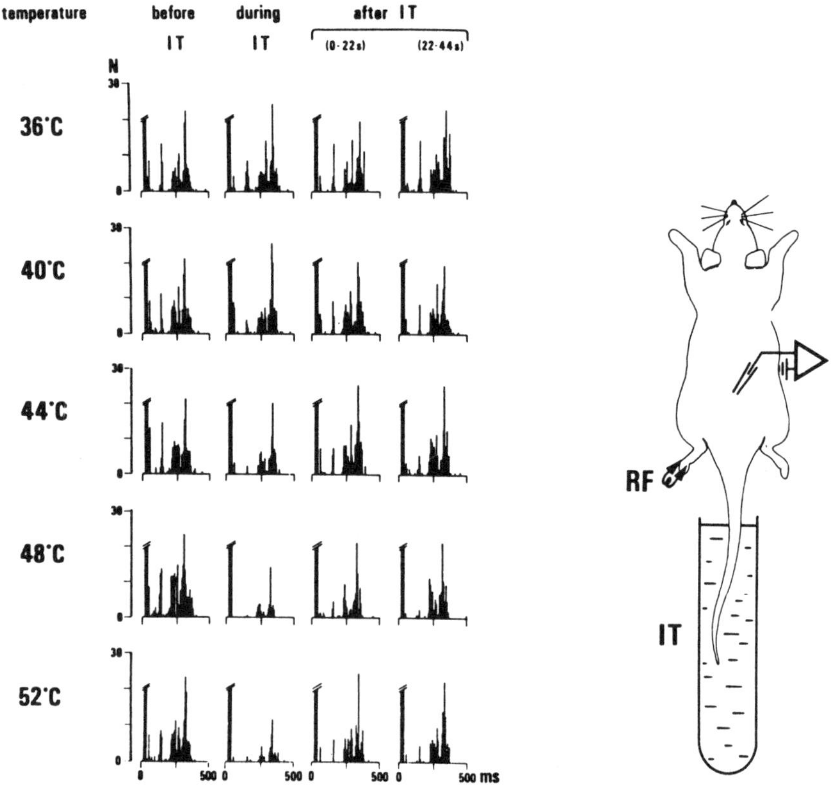

Figure 4.6 Effects of heating the tail to various temperatures, on the response of a convergent neurone to the suprathreshold electrical stimulation of its hindpaw receptive field (from Le Bars *et al.*, 1981a).

This neurone responded to Aα and C fibre inputs. Post-stimulus histograms (15 trials, bin width 5 ms) were obtained before, during and after immersion of the tail (IT) in a water bath (temperatures indicated on the left). Clear inhibitions of the C-fibre responses were observed for the highest temperatures.

propriospinal inhibitory mechanisms may also be triggered by noxious inputs (Gerhart *et al.*, 1981b; Fitzgerald, 1982). For example, in unanaesthetized spinal rats, some activities of convergent neurones (e.g. responses to sustained pinch) can be depressed to some extent by distant noxious stimuli (Cadden *et al.*, 1983). Unlike the diffuse noxious inhibitory controls observed in intact animals, these inhibitions appear to involve only some of the convergent neurones (roughly 50%). They are also weaker and return to base-line levels within 30 seconds. Furthermore, these inhibitory effects, although concerning several segments are more marked for noxious stimuli applied to structures proximal to the excitatory receptive field than for stimuli applied more distally.

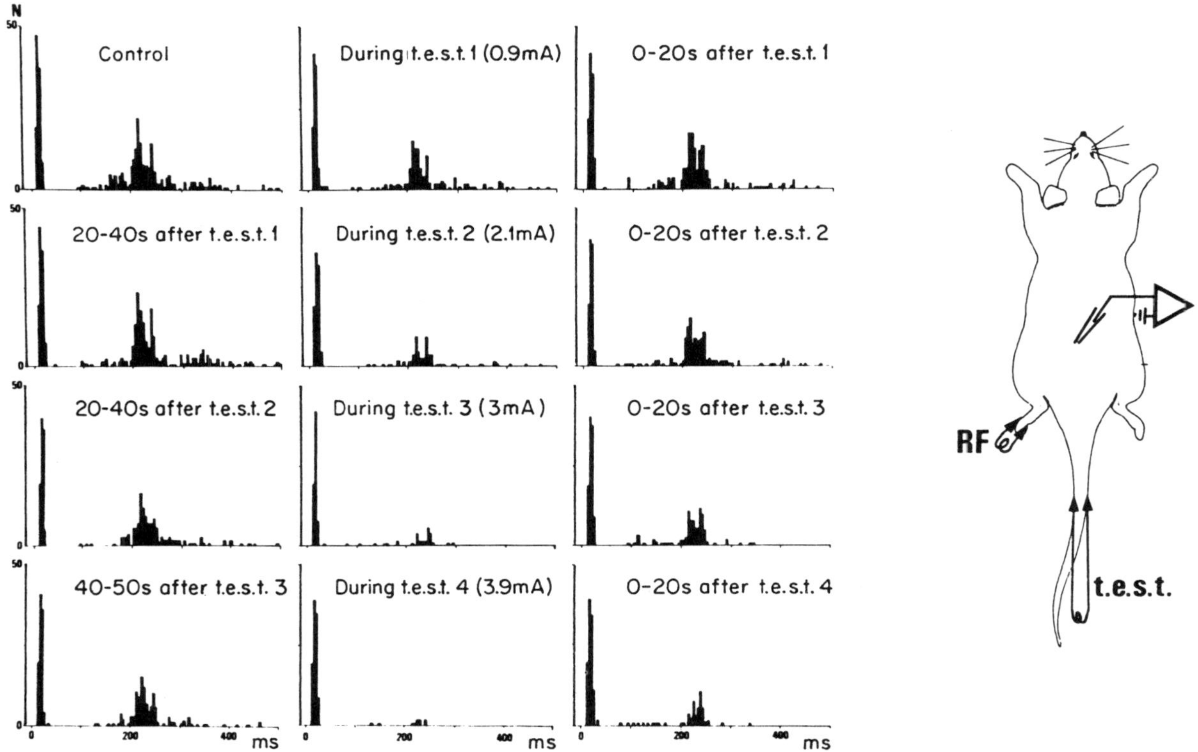

Figure 4.7 Effect of transcutaneous electrical stimulation of the tail (t.e.s.t. : 50 Hz, 1 ms width, 500 ms duration) on the response of a convergent neurone to suprathreshold electrical stimulation of its hindpaw receptive field (from Le Bars *et al.*, 1979a).

Post-stimulus histograms (20 trials, bin width 5 ms) were obtained before, during, and after the application of the conditioning stimulus (from left to right). Note that increasing the conditioning current intensity resulted in an increasing inhibition of the C-fibre responses.

For example, noxious stimuli applied to the tail or the contralateral hindpaw are much more effective in reducing responses of a neurone whose excitatory receptive field is located on the ipsilateral hindpaw than identical stimuli applied to the forepaw. The circuitry and pharmacology of such propriospinal inhibitory systems is, as yet, unknown.

(c) Mechanisms underlying diffuse noxious inhibitory controls

Since diffuse noxious inhibitory control is not demonstrable in anaesthetized animals with a cervical section of the spinal cord ('spinal animals') one can conclude that the underlying mechanisms are not confined to the spinal cord and involve pathways ascending from and descending to it. These controls appear to be clearly different from other controls triggered by somatic stimuli such as the segmental inhibitory controls triggered by innocuous inputs (see Section IIA), the propriospinal controls triggered by noxious inputs (see Section IIB(b)) and the heterosegmental and heterosensorial controls, described in chloralose and anaesthetized cats which, in addition to affecting convergent neurones affect neurones responding only to tactile stimuli (Besson and Rivot, 1972).

Due to the ascending/descending nature of the loop which originates from the peripheral nociceptors and sustains diffuse noxious inhibitory control, it has been postulated (Le Bars *et al.*, 1979b) that such controls involve structures, which when electrically stimulated induce profound analgesia. This is supported by the following evidence.

(a) *Descending control systems triggered by electrical stimulation of brainstem structures ('stimulation produced analgesia')*. It is well established (see references in Liebeskind *et al.*, 1976; Mayer and Price, 1976; Fields and Basbaum, 1978; Basbaum and Fields, 1978, 1980; Besson *et al.*, 1979, 1981; Mayer, 1979; Besson, 1980) that strong analgesia can be elicited by the electrical stimulation of brainstem structures such as the periaqueductal grey and certain raphé nuclei. These analgesic effects are most probably, at least in part, the result of the activation of descending inhibitory pathways which block the spinal transmission of nociceptive messages, especially those carried by convergent neurones. Periaqueductal grey stimulation induces strong inhibitory effects upon dorsal horn convergent neurones (Guilbaud *et al.*, 1972; Liebeskind *et al.*, 1973; Oliveras *et al.*, 1974; Carstens *et al.*, 1979, 1980, 1981a; Duggan and Griersmith, 1979; Hayes *et al.*, 1979) and such an action appears to be indirect since the periaqueductal grey has few spinal projections (Kuypers and Maisky, 1975; Basbaum and Fields, 1979; Tohyama *et al.*, 1979; Bowker *et al.*, 1981). On the basis of both anatomical (Ruda, 1975; Taber-Pierce *et al.*, 1976; Gallager and Pert, 1978; Abols and Basbaum, 1981) and electrophysiological evidence (Fields and Anderson, 1978; Lovick *et al.*, 1978a, b;

Behbehani and Fields, 1979; Pomeroy and Behbehani, 1979; Shan and Dostrovsky, 1980), it is generally accepted that the spinal inhibitory effects induced by stimulation of the periaqueductal grey result from the activation of the nucleus raphé magnus. Furthermore, electrical stimulation of this nucleus induces both stronger analgesic effects than those originating from the periaqueductal grey (Oliveras *et al.*, 1975, 1979) and important depressions of the activity of convergent neurones (Basbaum *et al.*, 1976; Beall *et al.*, 1976; Le Bars *et al.*, 1976; Fields *et al.*, 1977; Guilbaud *et al.*, 1977; Willis *et al.*, 1977; Belcher *et al.*, 1978; Duggan and Griersmith, 1979; McCreery *et al.*, 1979; Menetrey *et al.*, 1980; Rivot *et al.*, 1979, 1980; Gerhart *et al.*, 1981a; Iggo *et al.*, 1981).

(b) *Involvement of 5HT bulbospinal pathways in diffuse noxious inhibitory controls* The nucleus raphé magnus projects massively and directly towards the spinal cord (Brodal *et al.*, 1960; Basbaum *et al.*, 1976, 1978; Kneisley *et al.*, 1978; Leichnetz *et al.*, 1978; Martin *et al.*, 1978; Basbaum and Fields, 1979; Tohyama *et al.*, 1979; Zemlan and Pfaff, 1979; Watkins *et al.*, 1980) and is partly serotonergic (Dahlström and Fuxe, 1965; Oliveras *et al.*, 1977). These fibres travel through the dorsolateral funiculus which when sectioned counteracts the inhibitory effects induced on dorsal horn neurones by raphé magnus stimulation (Basbaum *et al.*, 1976; Fields *et al.*, 1977; Willis *et al.*, 1977). Such inhibitory effects are also reduced in animals pretreated with the inhibitor of serotonin synthesis, *p*-chlorophenylalanine (Rivot *et al.*, 1980). In addition, microelectrophoretic application of 5HT induces a depression of dorsal horn neuronal responses to noxious inputs (Randić and Yu, 1976; Belcher *et al.*, 1978; Headley *et al.*, 1978; Jordan *et al.*, 1978, 1979; Griersmith and Duggan, 1980) and these effects are particularly clear when 5HT is applied within the superficial layers of the dorsal horn where dense 5HT terminals have been found (Ruda and Gobel, 1980).

All together these data tend to suggest that stimulation of the nucleus raphé magnus exerts its inhibitory effects by releasing 5HT within the dorsal horn. This has actually been demonstrated (Rivot *et al.*, 1982). Indeed, when 5HT is injected intrathecally, hypoalgesia ensues (Wang, 1977; Yaksh and Wilson, 1979). Further evidence of the involvement of 5HT pathways in inhibitory controls comes from a number of different approaches.

(i) *Electrolytic lesions of nucleus raphé magnus (Dickenson et al., 1980b).* Diffuse noxious inhibitory controls were studied during recordings of neurones before and after electrolytic lesions of the nucleus raphé magnus. When the lesion included the whole nucleus then the inhibitory effects were strongly reduced whereas partial lesions resulted in less severe impairments in their strength.

(ii) *5HT depletion (Dickenson et al., 1981).* Diffuse noxious inhibitory controls in animals pretreated with *p*-chlorophenylalanine were found to be strongly reduced in comparison with control animals. For instance, inhibitory effects observed at the lumbar level, induced by intraperitoneal injection of bradykinin, tail pinch, muzzle pinch, or noxious heat applied on the tail, were respectively reduced by 47%, 63%, 87%, and 63% in the pretreated animals. Note that the effects did not disappear even though there was an essentially total depletion of 5HT in the spinal cord. This suggests that additional and complementary mechanisms are implicated. In fact, in *p*-chlorophenylalanine pretreated animals, the inhibitory effects of the above noxious stimuli were very variable and in some cases even facilitatory effects were observed.

(iii) *Blockade of 5HT receptors (Chitour et al., 1982).* Two 5HT receptor blockers (cinanserin and metergoline) strongly depressed diffuse noxious inhibitory control. This is illustrated in Figure 4.8, where noxious heat applied to the tail and noxious pinch on the nose were the stimuli.

(iv) *Increase of 5HT synthesis (Chitour et al., 1982).* As shown in Figure 4.9

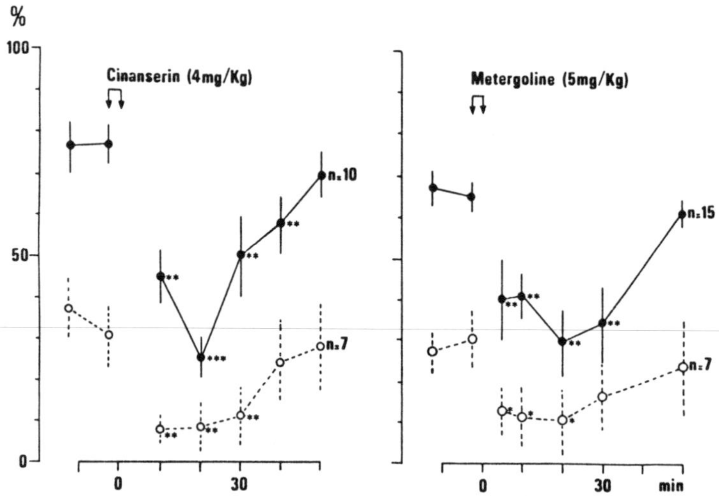

FIGURE 4.8 Time course of the effect of intravenously injected cinanserin (left) or metergoline (right) upon diffuse noxious inhibitory controls (from Chitour *et al.*, 1982).

The ordinates indicate the percentage inhibitions during the application of the noxious stimulus (left: immersion of the tail in a 52°C water bath; right: pinch of the nose) upon the C-fibre responses (solid line) and the Aα-fibre responses (broken line), induced by electrical stimulation of a hindpaw extremity. Note that both 5-HT receptor blockers had similar effects on the inhibitions of both types of neuronal response.

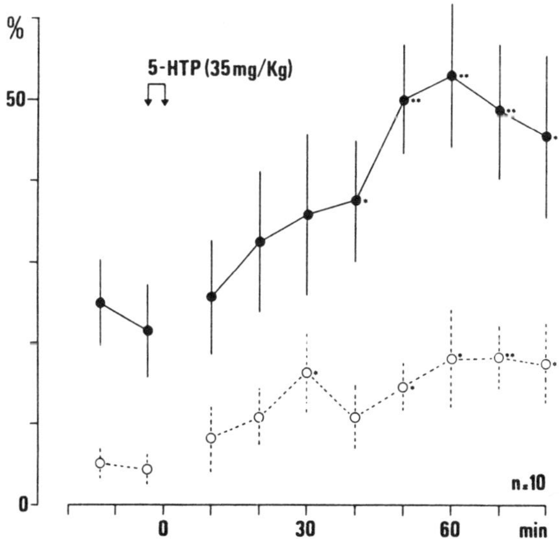

Figure 4.9 Time course of the effect of intravenously injected 5-HTP upon diffuse noxious inhibitory control triggered by a moderate noxious stimulus (immersion of the tail in 46–48 °C water bath) (from Chitour *et al.*, 1982).

Symbols as in Figure 4.8. Note that the precursor of serotonin synthesis induced a progressive increase in the inhibition of both the C-fibre responses (solid line) and the Aα-fibre responses (dotted line) elicited from a hindpaw extremity. Note also that the apparent maximal effect was one hour after the injection.

the systemic administration of 5-hydroxytryptophan, the precursor of 5HT synthesis, was found to potentiate diffuse noxious inhibitory controls.

Taken together, these data provide evidence for the hypothesis that diffuse noxious inhibitory controls are mediated, at least in part, via the bulbo-spinal serotonergic system. Indeed, spinal 5HT only occurs in terminals of neurones, the somata being located in supraspinal structures (Dahlström and Fuxe, 1965; Magnusson, 1973; Stanton *et al.*, 1975; Oliveras *et al.*, 1977). The superficial layers of the dorsal horn are rich in 5HT binding sites (Young and Kuhar, 1980) and contain 5HT terminals which synapse with dendrites of dorsal horn neurones (Ruda and Gobel, 1980; Ruda *et al.*, 1981). In addition, as previously mentioned, convergent neurones can be inhibited by the microelectrophoretic application of 5HT (Randić and Yu, 1976; Belcher *et al.*, 1978; Jordan *et al.*, 1978, 1979; Headley *et al.*, 1978; Griersmith and Duggan, 1980).

Parallelism between inhibitions mediated by the nucleus raphé magnus or by diffuse noxious controls is not only suggested by the experiments using raphé magnus lesions but also by those using *p*-chlorophenylalanine. In control animals, almost all convergent neurones are strongly inhibited both by heterotopic noxious stimuli and by electrical stimulation of the raphé magnus. These effects are similarly reduced by *p*-chlorophenylalanine (Rivot *et al.*, 1980; Dickenson *et al.*, 1981).

On the other hand, the unambiguous effects of 5HT receptor blockers against diffuse noxious inhibitory controls contrast with their, on the whole, slight effects on the inhibitory action of raphé magnus stimulation (Belcher *et al.*, 1978; Besson, 1980; Griersmith *et al.*, 1981). This apparent contradiction could be explained by the fact that raphé stimulation activates all the local neuronal elements, whether serotonergic or not, in an artificial and synchronized manner. In the face of a 5HT block, parallel systems may take over. In this respect it is worth pointing out that inhibitory effects induced on dorsal horn convergent neurones by periaqueductal grey stimulation are reduced by 5HT antagonists (Guildbaud *et al.*, 1973; Carstens *et al.*, 1981b). It seems therefore that the bulbo-spinal 5HT control of these neurones can be blocked by 5HT antagonists, but only when such a control is indirectly triggered.

Nevertheless, neurochemical experiments clearly demonstrate that bulbo-spinal 5HT systems can be activated by raphé stimulation (Bourgoin *et al.*, 1980; Rivot *et al.*, 1982) and the same systems are probably activated by noxious peripheral inputs. Indeed, the bilateral stimulation of the sciatic nerve, in the cat, with current intensities high enough to recruit A and/or C fibres induced the release of 5HT within the subarachnoid space, and this effect disappeared during thoracic cold block (Tyce and Yaksh, 1981). In addition, noxious stimulation of the tail induces a larger increase of 5HT synthesis in the dorsal than in the central horn (Weil-Fugazza *et al.*, 1981). These data are in keeping with the elevated concentrations of 5-hydroxyindoleacetic acid in the lumbar cerebrospinal fluid of patients suffering from chronic or acute pain (Ghia *et al.*, 1981).

(c) *Involvement of endogenous opiates.* The parallelism between the consequences of raphé magnus stimulation and the activation of diffuse noxious inhibitory controls is further substantiated by their similar susceptibilities to naloxone. Figure 4.10 shows that in the rat 0.3 mg/kg naloxone given intravenously depresses the inhibitory controls by 40–50% (Le Bars *et al.*, 1981c). Very similar reductions are achieved in the same species with equivalent doses following raphé magnus stimulation (Rivot *et al.*, 1979).

As naloxone was administered systematically, it is difficult to reach conclusions as to the target responsible for the effects we have described. From the localization of enkephalinergic interneurones, naloxone might have been

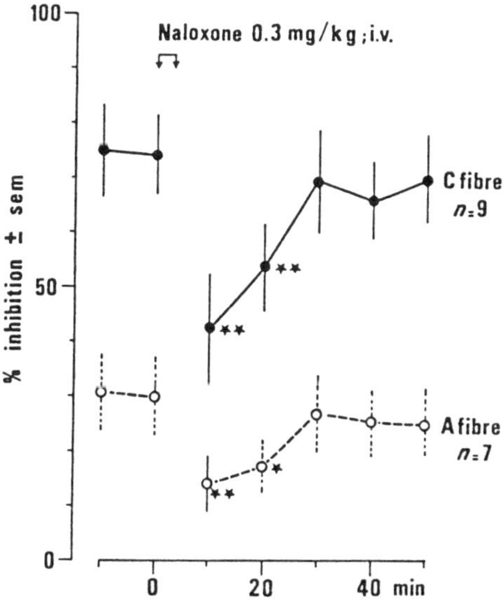

FIGURE 4.10 Time course of the effect of naloxone upon diffuse noxious inhibitory control triggered by immersion of the tail in a 52°C water bath (from Le Bars *et al.*, 1981c).

Symbols as in Figure 4.8. Note that the opiate antagonist transiently reduced the inhibitions of both the C-fibre responses (solid line) and the Aα-fibre responses (dotted line) elicited from a hindpaw extremity.

active at supraspinal and/or spinal sites. An effect of naloxone on the raphé magnus is consistent with its richness in enkephalin-containing interneurones (Hökfelt *et al.*, 1977; Sar *et al.*, 1978). In addition, a spinal target for naloxone is highly probable since the superficial layers of the dorsal horn are also rich in enkephalin-containing terminals (Hökfelt *et al.*, 1977; Simantov *et al.*, 1977; Sar *et al.*, 1978; Seybold and Elde, 1980; Aronin *et al.*, 1981; Hunt *et al.*, 1980, 1981; Glazer and Basbaum, 1981) and opiate receptors (Atweh and Kuhar, 1977).

Since naloxone is a relatively specific opiate antagonist, at least in low doses (see Goldstein, 1979), these data suggest the participation of endorphins (most probably the enkephalins) in diffuse noxious inhibitory control. However, it should be noted that the analgesic effect of intrathecal 5HT is not blocked by naloxone (Yaksh and Wilson, 1979).

(d) *End-point mechanisms of inhibition*. We have emphasized that diffuse noxious inhibitory controls affect all activities of convergent neurones; i.e. the neuronal responses to the activation of both A and C peripheral fibres. In addition several pharmacological agents (cinanserin, metergoline, naloxone), all alter the inhibitions in a similar way whether they concern the responses to one or the other group of fibres (see Figures 4.8, 4.9, 4.10). These properties strongly suggest that a final post-synaptic mechanism is responsible for the inhibitions. This is also suggested by the fact that inhibitory controls strongly depress convergent neurone excitation induced by direct microelectrophoretic application of glutamic acid (Villanueva *et al.*, 1982). Since glutamate directly excites the neuronal membrane (Curtis and Watkins, 1960; Zieglgänsberger and Puil, 1973; Puil, 1981), it is most probable that membrane hyperpolarization is ultimately involved at this level. This further emphasizes the parallelism between diffuse noxious inhibitory controls and the inhibitions triggered by raphé magnus stimulation as such stimulation produces inhibitory post-synaptic potentials during the recording of convergent spinothalamic neurones (Giesler *et al.*, 1981). However, complementary presynaptic mechanisms cannot be excluded (e.g., see Proudfit and Anderson, 1974; Lovick *et al.*, 1978b; Hentall and Fields, 1979; Martin *et al.*, 1979).

III SUMMARY AND CONCLUSIONS

Electrophysiological data thus demonstrate that a noxious stimulus applied to a body area (e.g. the tail) triggers not only a chain of excitatory events but also (via a supraspinal loop) diffuse inhibitory processes involving all spinal and trigeminal convergent neurones not directly excited by the initial stimulus. As a noxious stimulus seems able to trigger certain brainstem structures and thus to inhibit convergent neurones, even though it is apparently perceived as painful, diffuse noxious inhibitory controls might be involved in nociception. Such a suggestion seems to be supported by the close correlation between the intensity of the stimulus and the strength of inhibitory effects (Le Bars *et al.*, 1981a, see Figures 4.6 and 4.7). The possibility of an encoding of nociceptive information by inhibitory processes can therefore be envisaged and is supported by the fact that diffuse noxious inhibitory controls affect nearly all spino- and trigeminothalamic convergent neurones (Dickenson and Le Bars, 1982).

As convergent neurones are not only activated by noxious inputs but also, to an appreciable degree by weak mechanical stimuli (Le Bars and Chitour, 1983), we have recently proposed (Le Bars *et al.*, 1979b) a model in which nociceptive reactions could be triggered by a contrast signal between excitatory information emanating from both the segmental pool of convergent and nociceptive-specific neurones and the diffuse noxious inhibitory control-mediated silencing of the remaining convergent neuronal population (Figure 4.11). The theoretical framework of such a hypothesis, including its possible relationship with morphine analgesia, has been developed elsewhere (Le Bars *et al.*, 1981b, 1982a,b). Such a functional role is supported by the paradoxical

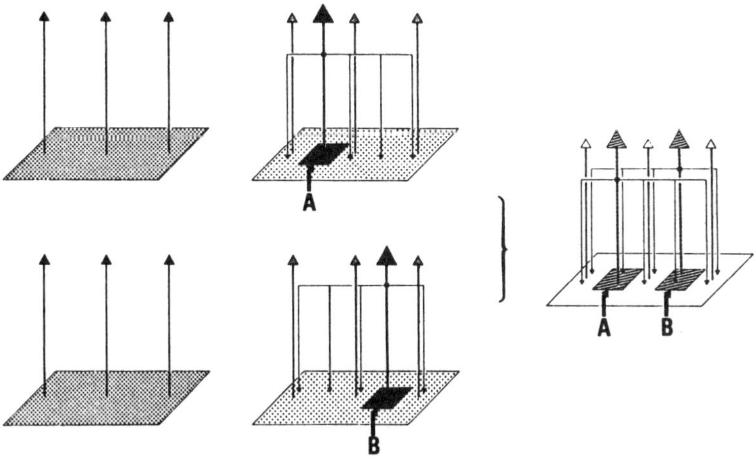

FIGURE 4.11 Hypothetical interpretation of the diffuse noxious inhibitory control system with reference to counter-irritation phenomena.

In the absence of noxious stimuli (left), the global activity (horizontal surface) of both spinal and trigeminal convergent neurones would be of a reasonably high order, sending a kind of 'noise' towards the brain (upwards arrows).

A noxious stimulus (A or B) activates both noxious and convergent segmental neurones, which send an excitatory signal to the brain (filled arrow); this input triggers the diffuse noxious inhibitory control system (downwards arrows) with a consequent reduction of the activity of the remaining non-segmental convergent units not directly affected by the initial stimulus. Hence, a contrast signal is set up between the activities of the two neuronal populations (upwards arrows).

In this model, the concurrent application of two noxious stimuli, i.e. A and B (right), would mutually influence the neuronal responses with the final output depending on the relative strengths of the stimuli.

observation of counter-irritation phenomena (see Section I). Referring to Figures 4.5, 4.6, or 4.7, we note that the response of a convergent neurone to noxious stimuli is highly depressed by the application of a second and stronger noxious stimuli applied on areas of the body remote from the excitatory receptive field of the neurone under study. If convergent neurones play an important role in the transmission of nociceptive messages, one could postulate that the concurrent application of two distinct noxious stimuli would result in attenuation of the pain resulting from the weaker stimulus. In such a system, the final sensation would depend not only on a balancing effect between two peripheral noxious inputs to the brain but also on the relative contribution of these inputs to the silencing of the background activity of convergent neurones (Figure 4.11, right). From the theoretical standpoint, the behavioural approach to this system in animal models is not easy to clearly define. As illustrated in Figure 4.4, each of the peripheral noxious stimuli might be considered as being either inhibitor or inhibited.

Further difficulties in this field arise from the fact that a noxious stimulus could trigger additional neurophysiological mechanisms which presumably have behavioural significance. For instance, electrical somatic stimulation, whether noxious or non-noxious, would most certainly trigger, via large diameter afferents, segmental inhibitory processes and noxious somatic stimulation would trigger propriospinal inhibitory processes in addition to diffuse noxious inhibitory controls (see Section IIB). Also, there is electrophysiological evidence (Willer and AlbeFessard, 1980) that stress itself —in the absence of pain sensations — induces a decrease of nociceptive reflexes in man.

These considerations emphasize the multiplicity of pain modulation systems which could be triggered by somatic reiterated stimuli and therefore, the possibility that one or other of these systems might predominate under specific experimental conditions. For instance, the distance between the points of application of the two stimuli (e.g., see Watkins *et al.*, 1982a) or the duration of the inhibition stimulus (e.g., see Lewis *et al.*, 1980) must be critical factors for consideration. The pharmacological manipulation of such multicomponent systems introduce additional complicating variables, while the diffuse nature of the control systems triggered by heterotopic noxious stimuli could also be a complicating factor. If one accepts the interpretation shown in Figure 4.11 (right) the results of pharmacological manipulations of such a system require consideration with respect to the effects of drugs not only on the neuronal responses to the two stimuli involved but also on the background activity of convergent neurones.

ACKNOWLEDGEMENTS

We wish to thank Mr H. de Pommery for the photography and Miss M. Hoch and Miss M. Cayla for secretarial help.

S. W. Cadden was supported by a Royal Society European Science Exchange Programme fellowship in conjunction with the Centre National de la Recherche Scientifique (CNRS).

L. Villanueva, on leave from the Department of Pharmacology of the University of Chile, was supported by a scholarship from the French government.

This work was supported by l'Institut National de la Santé et de la Recherche Médicale (INSERM), PRC no 120034 and CRL 82 60 29.

REFERENCES

Abols, I. A. and Basbaum, A. I. (1981). Afferent connections of the rostral medulla of the cat: a neural substrate for midbrain-medullary interactions in the modulation of pain. *J. Comp. Neurol.*, **201**, 285–297.

Adair, E. E., Stevens, J. C. and Marks, L. E. (1968). Thermally induced pain: the dol scale and the psychological power law. *Amer. J. Psychol.*, **81**, 147–164.

Anderson, K. V., Pearl, G. S. and Honeycutt, C. (1976). Behavioural evidence showing the predominance of diffuse pain stimuli over discrete stimuli in influencing perception. *J. Neurosci. Res.*, **2**, 283–289.

Aronin, N., Di Figlia, M., Liotta, A. S. and Martin, J. B. (1981). Ultrastructural localization and biochemical features of immunoreactive leu-enkephalin in monkey dorsal horn. *J. Neurosc.*, **1**, 561–577.

Atweh, S. F. and Kuhar, M. J. (1977). Autoradiographic localization of opiate receptors in rat brain. I—Spinal cord and lower medulla. *Brain Res.*, **124**, 53–67.

Basbaum, A. I., Clanton, C. H. and Fields, H. L. (1976). Opiate and stimulus produced analgesia: functional anatomy of a medullospinal pathway. *Proc. Natl Acad. Sci. (USA)*, **73**, 4685–4688.

Basbaum, A. I., Clanton, C. H. and Fields, H. L. (1978). Three bulbospinal pathways from the rostral medulla of the cat: an autoradiographic study of pain modulating systems. *J. Comp. Neurol.*, 209–224.

Basbaum, A. I. and Fields, H. L. (1978). Endogenous pain control mechanisms: review and hypothesis. *Annals Neurol.*, **4**, 451–462.

Basbaum, A. I. and Fields, H. L. (1979). The origin of descending pathways in the dorsolateral funiculus of the spinal cord of the cat and rat: further studies on the anatomy of pain modulation. *J. Comp. Neurol.*, **187**, 513–532.

Basbaum, A. I. and Fields, H. L. (1980). Pain control: a new role for the medullary reticular formation, in *The Reticular Formation Revisited* (eds J. A. Hobson and M. A. B. Brazier). Raven Press, New York, 329–348.

Beall, J. A., Martin, R. F., Applebaum, A. E. and Willis, W. D. (1976). Inhibition of primate spinothalamic tract neurons by stimulation in the region of nucleus raphé magnus. *Brain Res.*, **114**, 328–333.

Behbehani, M. M. and Fields, H. L. (1979). Evidence that an excitatory connection between the periaqueductal gray and nucleus raphé magnus mediates stimulation produced analgesia. *Brain Res.*, **170**, 85–93.

Belcher, G., Ryall, R. W. and Schaffner, R. (1978). The differential effects of 5-hydroxytryptamine, noradrenaline and raphé stimulation on nociceptive and non-nociceptive dorsal horn interneurons in the cat. *Brain Res.*, **151**, 307–321.

Berlin, L., Goodell, H. and Wolff, H. G. (1958). Studies on pain. Relation of pain perception and central inhibitory effect of noxious stimulation to phenomenon of extinction of pain. *Arch. Neurol. Psychiat. (Chicago)*, **80**, 533–543.

Besson, J. M. (1980). Supraspinal modulation of the segmental transmission of pain, in *Pain and Society*. (eds H. W. Kosterlitz and L. Y. Terenius), Dahlem Konferenzen, Weinheim Verlag Chemie, GmbH, 161–182.

Besson, J. M. and Rivot, J. P. (1972). Heterosegmental, heterosensory and cortical inhibitory effects on dorsal interneurones in the cat's spinal cord. *Elctroenceph. clin. Neurophysiol.*, **33**, 195–206.

Besson, J. M., Conseiller, C., Hammann, K. F. and Maillard, M. C. (1972). Modifications of dorsal horn cell activities in the spinal cord, after intra-arterial injection of bradykinin. *J. Physiol (Lond.)*, **221**, 189–205.

Besson, J. M., Catchlove, R. F. H., Feltz, P. and Le Bars, D. (1974). Further evidence for post-synaptic inhibitions on lamina V dorsal horn interneurons. *Brain Res.*, **66**, 531–536.

Besson, J. M., Dickenson, A. H., Le Bars, D. and Oliveras, J. L. (1979). Opiate analgesia: the physiology and pharmacology of spinal pain systems, in *Advances in Pharmacology and Therapeutics* (ed. C. Dumont), Neurosychopharmacology, vol. 5, Pergamon Press, Oxford, 61–81.

Besson, J. M., Oliveras, J. L., Chaouch, A. and Rivot, J. P. (1981). Role of the raphé nuclei in stimulation producing analgesia, in *Serotonin: Current Aspects of Neurochemistry and Function* (Eds B. Haber, S. Gabay, M. R. Issidorides, S. G. A. Alivisatos), Plenum Publishing Corporation, 153–176.

Besson, J. M., Guilbaud, G., Abdelmoumene, M. and Chaouch, A. (1982). Physiologie de la nociception. *J. Physiol. (Paris)*, **78**, 7–107.

Bodnar, R. J., Kordower, J. H., Wallace, M. M. and Tamir, H. (1981). Stress and morphine analgesia: alterations following *p*-chlorophenylalanine. *Pharmacol. Biochem. and Behavior*, **14**, 645–651.

Bourgoin, S., Oliveras, J. L., Bruxelle, J., Hamon, M. and Besson, J. M. (1980). Electrical stimulation of the nucleus raphé magnus in the rat. Effects on the 5-HT metabolism in the spinal cord. *Brain Res.*, **194**, 377–389.

Bowker, R. M., Steinbusch, H. W. M. and Coulter, J. D. (1981). Serotonergic and peptidergic projections to the spinal cord demonstrated by a combined retrograde HRP histochemical and immunocytochemical staining method. *Brain Res.*, **211**, 412–417.

Brodal, A., Taber, E. and Walberg, F. (1960). The raphé nuclei of the brain stem in the cat. II — Efferent connections. *J. Comp. Neurol.*, **114**, 239–259.

Brown, A. G., Hamann, W. C. and Martin, H. F. (1973). Interactions of cutaneous myelinated (A) and non-myelinated (C) fibres on transmission through the spinocervical tract. *Brain Res.*, **53**, 222–226.

Buckett, W. R. (1979). Peripheral stimulation in mice induces short-duration analgesia preventable by naloxone. *Europ. J. Pharmacol.*, **58**, 169–178.

Buckett, W. R. (1981). Pharmacological studies on stimulation-produced analgesia in mice. *Europ. J. Pharmacol.*, **69**, 281–290.

Cadden, S. W., Villanueva, L., Chitour, D. and Le Bars, D. (1983). Depression of activities of dorsal horn convergent neurones by propriospinal mechanisms triggered by noxious inputs; comparison with Diffuse Noxious Inhibitory Controls (DNIC). *Brain Res.*, **275**, 1–11.

Campbell, J. N. and Taub, A. (1973). Local analgesia from percutaneous electrical stimulation. A peripheral mechanism. *Arch Neurol. (Chicago)*, **28**, 347–350.

Carstens, E., Klumpp, D. and Zimmermann, M. (1979). The opiate antagonist, naloxone, does not affect descending inhibition from midbrain of nociceptive spinal neuronal discharges in the cat. *Neurosci. Lett.*, **11**, 723–727.

Carstens, E., Klumpp, D. and Zimmermann, M. (1980). Differential inhibitory effects of medial and lateral midbrain stimulation on spinal neuronal discharges to noxious skin heating in the cat. *J. Neurophysiol.*, **43**, 332–342.

Carstens, E., Bihl, H., Irvine, D. R. F. and Zimmermann, M. (1981a). Descending inhibitions from medial and lateral midbrain of spinal dorsal horn neuronal responses to noxious and non-noxious cutaneous stimuli in the cat. *J. Neurophysiol.*, **45**, 1029–1042.

Carstens, E., Fraunhoffer, M. and Zimmermann, M. (1981b). Serotonergic mediation of descending inhibition from midbrain periaqueductal gray, but not reticular formation, of spinal nociceptive transmission in the cat. *Pain*, **10**, 149–167.

Cervero, F. and Iggo, A. (1980). The substantia gelatinosa of the spinal cord. A critical review. *Brain*, **103**, 717–772.

Cervero, F., Iggo, A. and Ogawa, H. (1976). Nociceptor-driven dorsal horn neurons in the lumbar spinal cord of the cat. *Pain*, **2**, 5–24.

Chapman, D. B. and Way, L. E. (1982). Modification of endorphin/enkephalin analgesia and stress-induced analgesia by divalent cations, a cation chelator and an ionophore. *Br. J. Pharmacol.*, **75**, 389–396.

Cheser, G. B. and Chan, B. (1977). Footshock induced analgesia in mice: its reversal by naloxone and cross tolerance with morphine. *Life Sci.*, **21**, 1569–1574.

Chitour, D., Dickenson, A. H. and Le Bars, D. (1982). Pharmacological evidence for the involvement of serotonergic mechanisms in Diffuse Noxious Inhibitory Controls (DNIC). *Brain Res.*, **236**, 329–337.

Colpaert, F. C., Niemegeers, C. J. E. and Janssen, P. A. J. (1978). Nociceptive stimulation prevents development of tolerance to narcotic analgesia. *Europ. J. Pharmacol.*, **49**, 335–336.

Curtis, D. R. and Watkins, J. C. (1960). The excitation and depression of spinal neurones by structurally related amino acids. *J. Neurochem.*, **6**, 117–141.

Dahlström, A. and Fuxe, K. (1965). Evidence for the existence of monoamine neuron in the central nervous system. II — Experimentally induced changes in the intra-neuronal amine levels of the bulbospinal neuron system. *Acta Physiol. Scand.*, **64**, suppl. 247, 1–36.

Dickenson, A. H. and Le Bars, D. (1982). Diffuse noxious inhibitory controls (DNIC) involve trigemino thalamic and spinothalamic convergent neurones in the rat. *Exp. Brain Res.* **49**, 174–180.

Dickenson, A. H., Oliveras, J. L. and Besson, J. M. (1979). Role of the nucleus raphé magnus in opiate analgesia as studied by the microinjection technique in the rat. *Brain Res.*, **170**, 95–111.

Dickenson, A. H., Le Bars, D. and Besson, J. M. (1980a). Diffuse noxious inhibitory controls (DNIC). Effects on trigeminal nucleus caudalis neurones in the rat. *Brain Res.*, **200**, 293–305.

Dickenson, A. H., Le Bars, D. and Besson, J. M. (1980b). An involvement of nucleus raphé magnus in Diffuse Noxious Inhibitory Controls (DNIC). *Neurosci. Lett.* (suppl.), **5**, S375.

Dickenson, A. H., Rivot, J. P., Chaouch, A., Besson, J. M. and Le Bars, D. (1981). Diffuse noxious inhibitory controls (DNIC) in the rat with or without pCPA pretreatment. *Brain Res.*, **216**, 313–321.

De Niemeyer, F. (1869). *Traité de pathologie interne et de thérapeutique*, vol. II, Librairie Chamerot et Lauwereyns, Paris.

Duchenne de Boulogne (1855). *De l'électrisation localisée et de son application à la physiologie, à la pathologie et à la thérapeutique*. Baillière, Paris.

Duggan, A. W. and Griersmith, B. T. (1979). Inhibition of the spinal transmission of nociceptive information by supraspinal stimulation in the cat. *Pain*, **6**, 149–161.

Duncker, K. (1937). Some preliminary experiments on the mutual influence of pains. *Psychologische Forschung*, **21**, 311–326.

Eccles, J. C. and Krnjevic, K. (1959). Potential changes recorded inside primary afferent fibers within the spinal cord. *J. Physiol. (Lond.)*, **149**, 250–273.

Eccles, J. C., Schmidt, R. F. and Willis, W. D. (1963). Depolarisation of the central terminals of cutaneous afferent fibres. *J. Neurophysiol.*, **26**, 646–661.

Eriksson, M. B. E. and Sjölund, B. H. (1976). Acupuncturelike electroanalgesia in T.N.S.-resistant chronic pain, in *Sensory Functions of the Skin in Primates* (ed. Y. Zotterman), Pergamon Press, Oxford and New York, 575–581.

Fields, H. L. and Anderson, S. D. (1978). Evidence that raphé spinal neurons mediate opiate and midbrain stimulation produced analgesia. *Pain*, **5**, 333–349.

Fields, H. L. and Basbaum, A. E. (1978). Brain stem control of spinal pain transmission neurons. *Ann. Rev. Physiol.*, **40**, 193–221.

Fields, H. L., Basbaum, A. I., Clanton, C. H. and Anderson, S. D. (1977). Nucleus raphé magnus inhibition of spinal cord dorsal horn neurons. *Brain Res.*, **126**, 441–453.

Fitzgerald, M. (1982). The contralateral input to the dorsal horn of the spinal cord in the decerebrate spinal rat. *Brain Res.*, **236**, 275–287.

Foreman, R. D., Beall, J. E., Applebaum, A. E., Coulter, J. D. and Willis, W. D. (1976). Effects of dorsal column stimulation on primate spinothalamic tract neurons. *J. Neurophysiol.*, **39**, 534–546.

Fox, E. J. and Melzack, R. (1976a). Comparison of transcutaneous electrical stimulation and acupuncture in the treatment of chronic pain, in *Advances in Pain Research and Therapy*, (eds J. J. Bonica, D. Albe-Fessard), vol. 1, Raven Press, New York, 797–801.

Fox, E. J. and Melzack, R. (1976b). Transcutaneous electrical stimulation and acupuncture: comparison of treatment for low-back pain. *Pain,* **2**, 141–148.

Gallager, D. W. and Pert, A. (1978). Afferents to brain stem nuclei (brain stem raphé, nucleus reticularis pontis caudalis and nucleus gigantocellularis) in the rat as demonstrated by microiontophoretically applied horseradish peroxidase. *Brain Res.,* **144**, 257–276.

Gammon, G. D. and Starr, I. (1941). Studies on the relief of pain by counter-irritation. *J. Clin. Invest.,* **20**, 13–20,

Gerhart, K. D., Wilcox, T. K., Chung, J. M. and Willis, W. D. (1981a). Inhibition of nociceptive and non-nociceptive responses of primate spinothalamic cells by stimulation in medial brain stem. *J. Neurophysiol.,* **45**, 121–136.

Gerhart, K. D., Yezierski, R. P., Giesler, G. J. Jr. and Willis, W. D. (1981b). Inhibitory receptive field of primate spino-thalamic tract cells. *J. Neurophysiol.,* **46**, 1309–1325.

Ghia, J. N., Mueller, R. A., Duncan, G. H., Scott, D. S. and Mao, W. (1981). Serotonergic activity in man as a function of pain, pain mechanisms and depression. *Anesth. Analg. Curr. Res.,* **60**, 854–861.

Giesler, G. J. Jr., Gerhart, K. D., Yezierski, R. P., Wilcox, T. K. and Willis, W. D. (1981). Postsynaptic inhibition of primate spinothalamic neurons by stimulation in nucleus raphé magnus. *Brain Res.,* **204**, 184–188.

Glazer, E. J. and Basbaum, A. I. (1981). Immunohistochemical localization of Leucine-Enkephalin in the spinal cord of the cat: enkephalin-containing marginal neurons and pain modulation. *J. Comp. Neurol.,* **196**, 377–389.

Goldstein, A. (1979). Endorphins and pain: a critical review, in *Mechanisms of Pain and Analgesic Compounds* (eds R. F. Beers, Jr. E. G. Bassett), Raven Press, New York, 249–262.

Grant, A. E. (1964). Massage with ice (cryokinetics) in the treatment of painful conditions of the musculoskeletal pain. *Arch. of Phys. Med. and Rehab.,* **45**, 233–238.

Gregor, M. and Zimmermann, M. (1972). Characteristics of spinal neurones responding to cutaneous myelinated and unmyelinated fibres. *J. Physiol. (Lond.),* **221**, 555–576.

Griersmith, B. T. and Duggan A. W. (1980). Prolonged depression of spinal transmission of nociceptive information by 5-HT administered in the substantia gelatinosa: antagonism by methysergide. *Brain Res.,* **187**, 231–236.

Griersmith, B. T., Duggan, A. W. and North, R. A. (1981). Methysergide and supraspinal inhibition of the spinal transmission of nociceptive information in the anaesthetized cat. *Brain Res.,* **204**, 147–158.

Guilbaud, G., Besson, J. M., Liebeskind, J. C. and Oliveras, J. L. (1972). Analgésie induite par stimulation de la substance grise périaqueducale chez le chat: données comportementales et modifications de l'activité des interneurones de la corne dorsale de la moelle. *C. R. Acad. Sci., (Paris)*, **275**, 1055–1057.

Guilbaud, G., Besson, J. M., Oliveras, J. L. and Liebeskind, J. C. (1973). Suppression by LSD of the inhibitory effect exerted by dorsal raphé stimulation on certain spinal cord interneurons in the cat. *Brain Res.,* **61**, 417–422.

Guilbaud, G., Oliveras, J. L., Giesler, G. J. Jr. and Besson, J. M. (1977). Effects induced by stimulation of the centralis inferior nucleus of the raphé on dorsal horn interneurons in cat's spinal cord. *Brain Res.*, **126**, 355–360.

Gybels, J., Handwerker, H. O. and Van Hees, J. (1979). Comparison between the discharges of human nociceptive nerve fibres and the subject's rating of his sensation. *J. Physiol. (Lond.)*, **292**, 193–206.

Handwerker, H. O., Iggo, A. and Zimmermann, M. (1975). Segmental and supraspinal actions on dorsal horn neurons responding to noxious and non noxious skin stimuli. *Pain*, **1**, 147–165.

Hardy, J. D., Wolff, H. G. and Goodell, H. (1940). Studies on pain. A new method for measuring pain threshold: observations on spatial summation of pain. *J. Clin. Invest.*, **19**, 649–657.

Hardy, J. D., Goodell, H. and Wolff, H. G. (1951). The influence of skin temperature upon the pain threshold as evoked by thermal radiation. *Science*, **114**, 149–150.

Hayes, R. L., Bennett, G. J., Newlon, P. G. and Mayer, D. J. (1978). Behavioral and physiological studies of non-narcotic analgesia in the rat elicited by certain environmental stimuli. *Brain Res.*, **155**, 69–90.

Hayes, R. L., Price, D. D., Ruda, M. and Dubner, R. (1979). Suppression of nociceptive responses in the primate by electrical stimulation of the brain or morphine administration: behavioral and electrophysiological comparisons. *Brain Res.*, **167**, 417–421.

Hazouri, L. A. and Mueller, A. D. (1950). Pain threshold studies on paraplegic patients. *Arch. Neurol. Psychiat. (Chicago)*, **64**, 607–613.

Headley, P. M., Duggan, A. W. and Griersmith, B. T. (1978). Selective reduction by noradrenaline and 5-hydroxytryptamine of nociceptive responses of cat dorsal horn neurones. *Brain Res.*, **145**, 185–189.

Hentall, J. D. and Fields, H. L. (1979). Segmental and descending influences on intra-spinal thresholds of single C-fibers. *J. Neurophysiol.*, **42**, 1527–1537.

Hillman, P. and Wall. P. D. (1969). Inhibitory and excitatory factors influencing the receptive fields of lamina 5 spinal cord cells. *Exp. Brain Res.*, **9**, 284–306.

Hodge, C. J. (1972). Potential changes inside central afferent terminals secondary to stimulation of large- and small-diamater peripheral nerve fibers. *J. Neurophysiol.*, **35**, 30–43.

Hokfelt, T., Ljungdahl, A., Terenius, L., Elde, R. and Nilsson, G. (1977). Immunohistochemical analysis of peptide pathways possibly related to pain and analgesia: enkephalin and substance *P. Proc. Natl Acad. Sci. (USA)*, **74**, 3081–3085.

Hongo, T., Jankowska, E. and Lundberg, A. (1968). Post-synaptic excitation and inhibition from primary afferents in neurones of the spinocervical tract. *J. Physiol. (Lond.)*, **199**, 569–572.

Hunt, S. P., Kelly, J. S. and Emson, P. C. (1980). The electron microscopic localization of methionine-enkephaline within the superficial layers (I and II) of the spinal cord. *Neuroscience*, **5**, 1871–1890.

Hunt, S. P., Kelly, J. S., Emson, P. C., Kimmel, J. R., Miller, R. J. and Wu, H. Y. (1981). An immunohistochemical study of neuronal populations containing neuropeptides or γ-aminobutyrate within the superficial layers of the rat dorsal horn. *Neuroscience*, **6**, 1883–1898.

Hutson, P. H., Tricklebank, M. D. and Curzon, G. (1982). Enhancement of footshock-induced analgesia by spinal 5,7-dihydroxytryptamine lesions. *Brain Res.*, **237**, 367–372.

Iggo, A., McMillan, J. A. and Mokha, S. S. (1981). Modulation of spinal cord multireceptive neurones from locus coeruleus and nucleus raphé magnus in the cat. *J. Physiol. (Lond.)*, **319**, 107–108P.

Jeans, M. E. (1979). Relief of chronic pain by brief, intense transcutaneous electrical stimulation. A double-blind study. In (eds J. J. Bonica, J. C. Liebeskind and D. Albe-Fessard), *Advances in Pain Research and Therapy* vol. 3, Raven Press, New York, pp. 601–606.

Jordan, L. M., Kenshalo, D. R., Martin, R. F., Haber, L. H. and Willis, W. D. (1978). Depression of primate spinothalamic tract neurons by iontophoretic application of 5-hydroxytryptamine. *Pain,* **5**, 135–142.

Jordan, L. M., Kenshalo, D. R., Martin, R. F., Haber, L. H. and Willis, W. D. (1979). Two populations of spinothalamic tract neurons with opposite responses to 5-hydroxytryptamine. *Brain Res.,* **164**, 342–346.

Kane, K. and Taub, A. (1975). A history of local electrical analgesia. *Pain,* **1**, 125–138.

Koketsu, K. (1956). Intracellular potential changes of primary afferent nerve fibres in spinal cords of cats. *J. Neurophysiol.,* **19**, 375–392.

Kraus, E., Le Bars, D. and Besson, J. M. (1981). Behavioral confirmation of "Diffuse Noxious Inhibitory Controls" (DNIC) and evidence for a role of endogenous opiates. *Brain Res.,* **206**, 495–499.

Kraus, E., Besson, J. M. and Le Bars, D. (1982). Behavioural model for Diffuse Noxious Inhibitory Controls (DINC): potentiation by 5-hydroxytryptophan. *Brain Res.,* **231**, 461–465.

Kneisley, L. W., Bider, M. P. and Lavail, H. H. (1978). A study of the origin of brain stem projections to monkey spinal cord using the retrograde transport method. *Exp. Neurol.,* **60**, 116–139.

Kuypers, H. G. J. M. and Maisky, V. A. (1975). Retrograde transport of horseradish peroxidase from spinal cord to brain stem cell groups in the cat. *Neurosc. Letters,* **1**, 9–14.

Lamotte, R. H. and Campbell, J. N. (1978). Comparison of responses of warm and nociceptive C fiber afferent in monkey with human judgments of thermal pain. *J. Neurophysiol.,* **41**, 509–528.

Le Bars, D. and Chitour, D. (1983). Do convergent neurones in the spinal cord discriminate nociceptive from non-nociceptive information? *Pain*, **17**, 1–19.

Le Bars, D., Menetrey, D. and Besson, J. M. (1976). Effects of morphine upon the lamina V type cells activities in the dorsal horn of decerebrate cat. *Brain Res.,* **113**, 293–310.

Le Bars, D., Dickenson, A. H. and Besson, J. M. (1979a]. Diffuse Noxious Inhibitory Controls (DNIC). I — Effects on dorsal horn convergent neurones in the rat. *Pain,* **6**, 283–304.

Le Bars, D., Dickenson, A. H. and Besson, J. M. (1979b). Diffuse Noxious Inhibitory Controls (DNIC). II — Lack of effect on non-convergent neurones, supraspinal involvement and theoretical implications. *Pain,* **6**, 305–327.

Le Bars, D., Chitour, D. and Clot, A. M. (1981a). The encoding of thermal stimuli by Diffuse Noxious Inhibitory Controls (DNIC). *Brain Res.,* **230**, 394–399.

Le Bars, D., Chitour, D., Kraus, E., Clot, A. M., Dickenson, A. H. and Besson, J. M. (1981b). The effect of systemic morphine upon Diffuse Noxious Inhibitory Controls (DNIC) in the rat: evidence for a lifting of certain descending inhibitory controls of dorsal horn convergent neurones. *Brain Res.,* **215**, 257–274.

Le Bars, D., Chitour, D., Kraus, E., Dickenson, A. H. and Besson, J. M. (1981c). Effect of naloxone upon Diffuse Noxious Inhibitory Controls (DNIC) in the rat. *Brain Res.,* **204**, 387–402.

Le Bars, D., Dickenson, A. H. and Besson, J. M. (1982a). The triggering of bulbo-spinal serotonergic inhibitory controls by noxious peripheral inputs, in *Brainstem Control of Spinal Mechanisms*, (eds B. Sjölund, A. Björklund) pp. 381–410, Elsevier Biomedical Press.

Le Bars, D., Dickenson, A. H. and Besson, J. M. (1982b). Opiate analgesia and descending inhibitory controls systems, in *Advances in Pain Research and Therapy*, vol. 5, (eds U. Lindblom *et al.*), Raven Press, New York 341–372.

Le Bars, D., Roby, A. and Willer, J. C. (1983). Effects of heterotopic thermal stimuli on a nociceptive flexion reflex and the related pain sensation in man. *J. Physiol. (London)* **336**, 31.

Leichnetz, G. R., Watkins, L., Griffin, G., Martin, R. and Mayer, D. J. (1978). The projection from nucleus raphé magnus and other brain stem nuclei to the spinal cord in the rat: a study using HRP blue reaction. *Neurosc. Letters,* **8**, 119–124.

Levine, J. D., Gormley, J. and Fields, H. L. (1976). Observations on the analgesic effects of needle puncture (acupuncture). *Pain,* **2**, 149–159.

Lewis, J. W., Cannon, J. T. and Liebeskind, J. C. (1980). Opiod and non-opoid mechanisms of stress analgesia. *Science*, **208** 623–625.

Lewis, J. W., Sherman, J. E. and Liebeskind, J. C. (1981). Opioid and non-opioid stress analgesia: assessment of tolerance and cross-tolerance with morphine. *J. Neurosci.*, **4**, 358–363.

Liebeskind, J. C., Guilbaud, G., Besson, J. M. and Oliveras, J. L. (1973). Analgesia from electrical stimulation of the periaqueductal gray matter in the cat: behavioral observations and inhibitory effects on spinal cord interneurons. *Brain Res.*, **50**, 441–446.

Libeskind, J. C., Giesler, G. J. Jr. and Urca, G. (1976) Evidence pertaining to an endogenous mechanism of pain inhibition in the central nervous system, in *Sensory Functions of the Skin in Primates* (ed. I. Zotterman), Pergamon Press, Oxford, 561–573.

Lindblom, U., Tapper, D. N. and Wiesenfeld, Z. (1977). The effect of dorsal horn column stimulation on the noniceptive response of dorsal horn cells and its relevance to pain suppression. *Pain,* **4**, 133–144.

Long, D. M. and Hagfors, N. (1975). Electrical stimulation in the nervous system: the current status of electrical stimulation of the nervous system for relief of pain. *Pain,* **1**, 109–123.

Lovick, T. A., West, D. C. and Wolstencroft, H. H. (1978a). Responses of raphé spinal and other bulbar raphé neurones to stimulation of the periaqueductal gray in the cat. *Neurosc. Letters,* **8**, 45–49.

Lovick, T. A., West, D. C. and Wolstencroft, H. H. (1978b). A presynaptic action of the raphé on tooth pulp fibre terminals; is this mediated by an opioid peptide? In *Characteristics and Functions of Opioides* (eds J. M. Van Ree, L. Terenius, eds., Elsevier/ North-Holland, Amsterdam, 175–177.

McCreery, D. B., Bloedel, J. R. and Hames, E. G. (1979). Effects of stimulating in raphé nuclei and in reticular formation on response of spinothalamic neurons to mechanical stimuli. *J. Neurophysiol.*, **42**, 166–182.

Magnusson, T. (1973). Effect of chronic transection on dopamine, noradrenaline and 5-hydroxytroptamine in the rat spinal cord. *Naunyn-Schmiedeberg's Arch. Pharmac.*, **278**, 13–22.

Mann, F. (1974). Acupuncture analgesia, report of 100 experiments. *Brit. J. Anaesth.*, **46**, 361–364.

Martin, R. F., Haber, L. H. and Willis, W. D. (1979). Primary afferent depolarization of identified cutaneous fibers following stimulation in medial brain stem. *J. Neurophysiol.*, **42**, 779–790.

Martin, R. F., Jordan, L. M. and Willis, W. D. (1978). Differential projections of cat medullary raphé neurons demonstrated by retrograde labelling following spinal cord lesions. *J. Comp. Neurol.*, **182**, 77–88.

Mayer, D. J. (1979). Endogenous analgesia systems: neural and behavioral mechanisms, in *Advances in Pain Research and Therapy* (eds J. J. Bonica, J. C. Liebeskind, and D. Albe-Fessard, vol. 3, Raven Press, New York, 385–410.

Mayer, D. J. and Price, D. D. (1976). Central nervous system mechanisms of analgesia. *Pain,* **2**, 379–404.

Melzack, R. (1975). Prolonged relief of pain by brief, intense transcutaneous somatic stimulation. *Pain,* **1**, 357–373.

Melzack, R. and Wall, P. D. (1965). Pain mechanism: a new theory. *Science,* **150**, 971–979.

Melzack, R., Stillwell, D. M. and Fox, E. J. (1977). Trigger points and acupuncture points for pain: correlations and implications. *Pain,* **3**, 3–24.

Melzack, R., Guite, S. and Gonshor, A. (1980a). Relief of dental pain by ice massage of the hand. *Canad. Med. Ass. J.,* **122**, 189–191.

Melzack, R., Jeans, M. E., Stratford, J. G. and Monks, R. C. (1980b). Ice massage and transcutaneous electrical stimulation: comparison of treatment for low-back pain. *Pain,* **9**, 209–317.

Mendell, L. M. (1966). Physiological properties of unmyelinated fiber projections to the spinal cord. *Exp. Neurol.,* **16**, 316–332.

Menetrey, D., Chaouch, A. and Besson, J. M. (1980). Location and properties of dorsal horn neurons at origin of spinoreticular tract in lumbar enlargement of the rat. *J. Neurophysiol.,* **44**, 862–877.

Mennell, J. M. (1975). The therapeutic use of cold. *J. Amer. Osteopath. Ass.,* **74**, 1146–1158.

Merskey, H. and Evans, P. R. (1975). Variation in pain complaint threshold in psychiatric and neurological patients with pain. *Pain,* **1**, 73–79.

Meyer, G. A. and Fields, H. L. (1972). Causalgia treated by selective large fibres stimulation of peripheral nerve. *Brain,* **95**, 163–168.

Nashold, B. S. and Friedman, H. (1972). Dorsal column stimulation for control of pain. Preliminary report on 30 patients. *J. Neurosurg.,* **36**, 590–597.

Nathan, P. W. (1976). The gate-control theory of pain: a critical review. *Brain,* **99**, 123–158.

Nathan, P. W. and Wall, P. D. (1974). Treatment of post-herpetic neuralgia by prolonged electrical stimulation. *Brit. Med. J.,* **3**, 645–647.

Nielseon, K. D., Adams, J. E. and Hosobuchi, Y. (1975). Phantom limb pain. Treatment with dorsal column stimulation. *J. Neurosurg.,* **42**, 301–307.

Niemegeers, C. J. E., Van Bruggen, J. A. A. and Janssen, P. A. J. (1975). Suprofen, a potent antagonist of acetic acid-induced writhing in rat. *Arzneim. Forsch.,* **25**, 1505–1509.

Oliveras, J. L., Besson, J. M., Guilbaud, G. and Liebeskind, J. C. (1974). Behavioral and electrophysiological evidence of pain inhibition from midbrain stimulation in the cat. *Exp. Brain Res.,* **20**, 32–44.

Oliveras, J. L., Redjemi, F., Guilbaud, G. and Besson, J. M. (1975). Analgesia induced by electrical stimulation of the inferior centralis nucleus of the raphé in the cat. *Pain,* **1**, 139–145.

Oliveras, J. L., Bourgoin, S., Hery, F., Besson, J. M. and Hamon, M. (1977). The topographical distribution of serotoninergiv terminals in the spinal cord of the cat: biochemical mapping by combined use of microdissection and microassay procedures. *Brain Res.*, **138**, 393–406.

Oliveras, J. L., Guilbaud, G., and Besson, J. M. (1979). A map of serotoninergic structures involved in stimulation producing analgesia in unrestrained freely moving cats. *Brain Res.*, **164**, 317–322.

Parsons, C. M. and Goetzl, F. R. (1945). Effect of induced pain on theshold. *Proc. Soc. exp. Biol., (N.Y.)*, **60**, 327–329.

Pomeroy, S. L. and Behbehani, M. M. (1979). Physiological evidence for a projection from periacqueductal gray to nucleus raphe magnus, in the rat. *Brain Res.,* **176**, 143–147.

Price, D. D. and Wagman, I. H. (1970). The physiological roles of A and C fiber inputs to the dorsal horn of M. mulatta. *Exp. Neurol.,* **29**, 373–390.

Price, D. D., Hull, C. D., and Buchwald, N. A. (1971). Intracellular responses of dorsal horn cells to cutaneous and sural nerve A and C fiber stimuli. *Exp. Neurol.,* **33**, 291–309.

Proudfit, H. K. and Anderson, E. G. (1974). New long latency bulbospinal evoked potentials blocked by serotonin antagonists. *Brain Res.*, **65**, 542–546.

Puil, E. (1981). S-glutamate: its interactions with spinal neurons. *Brain Res. Reviews,* **3**, 229–322.

Randic, M. and Yu, H. H. (1976). Effects of 5-hydroxytryptamine and bradykinin in cat dorsal horn neurones activated by noxious stimuli. *Brain Res.,* **111**, 197–203.

Rexed, B. (1952). The cytoarchitectonic organization of the spinal cord in the cat. *J. Comp. Neurol.,* **96**, 415–496.

Rexed, B. (1954). A cytoarchitectonic atlas of the spinal cord in the cat. *J. Comp. Neurol.,* **100**, 297–380.

Rivot, J. P., Chaouch, A. and Besson, J. M. (1979). The influence of naloxone on the C-fiber response of dorsal horn neurons and their inhibitory control by raphé magnus stimulation. *Brain Res.,* **176**, 355–364.

Rivot, J. P., Chaouch, A. and Besson, J. M. (1980). Nucleus raphé magnus modulation of response of rat dorsal horn neurons to unmyelinated fiber inputs: partial involvement of serotonergic pathways. *J. Neurophysiol.,* **44**, 1039–1057.

Rivot, J. P., Chiang, C. Y. and Besson, J. M. (1982). Increase of serotonin metabolism within the dorsal horn of the spinal cord during nucleus raphé magnus stimulation, as revealed by in vivo electrochemical detection. *Brain Res.* **238**, 117–126.

Ruda, M. A. (1975). Autoradiographic study of the efferent projections of the midbrain central gray in the cat. *Anat. Rec.,* **181**, 468–469.

Ruda, M. A. and Gobel, S. (1980). Ultrastructural characterization of axonal endings in the substantia gelatinosa which take up (^{3}H) serotonin. *Brain Res.,* **184**, 57–83.

Ruda, M. A., Allen, B. and Gobel, S. (1981). Ultrastructural analysis of medial brain stem afferents to the superficial dorsal horn. *Brain Res.,* **205**, 175–180.

Sar, M., Stumpf, W. E., Miller, R. J., Chang, K. J. and Cuatrecasas, P. (1978). Immunohistochemical localization of enkephalin in rat brain and spinal cord. *J. Comp. Neurol.,* **182**, 17–38.

Sarlandière (1825). *Mémoire sur l'électro-acupuncture.* Paris.

Satran R. and Goldstein, M. N. (1973). Pain perception: modification of threshold of intolerance and cortical potentials by cutaneous stimulation. *Science,* **180**, 1201–1202.

Seybold, V. and Elde, R. (1980). Immunohistochemical studies of peptidergic neurons in the dorsal horn of the spinal cord. *J. Histochem. Cytochem.,* **28**, 367–370.

Shah, Y. and Dostrovsky, J. O. (1980). Electrophysiological evidence for a projection of the periaqueductal gray matter to nucleus raphé magnus in a cat and rat. *Brain Res.,* **193**, 534–538.

Shealy, C. N., Mortimer, J. T. and Hagfors, N. R. (1970). Dorsal column electroanalgesia. *J. Neurosurg.,* **32**, 560–564.

Simantov, R., Kuhar, M. J., Uhl, G. R. and Snyder, S. H. (1977). Opioid peptide enkephalin: immunohistochemical mapping in the rat central nervous system. *Proc. Natl Acad. Sci., USA,* **74**, 2167–2171.

Stanton, E. S., Smolen, P. M., Nashold, B. S. Jr., Dreyer, D. A. and Davis, J. N. (1975). Segmental analysis of spinal cord monoamines after thoracic transection in the dog. *Brain Res.,* **89**, 93–98.

Sternbach (1976). Psychological factors in Pain, in *Advances in Pain Research and Therapy*, vol. 1, (eds J. J. Bonica and D. Albe-Fessard) Raven Press, New York, pp. 293–299.

Syme, J. (1863). *The Principles of Surgery*, 5th ed., Murray, London.

Taber-Pierce, E. T., Foote, W. E., and Hobson, J. S. (1976). The efferent connections of the nucleus raphé dorsalis. *Brain Res.,* **107**, 137–144.

Tohyama, M., Sakai, K., Touret, M., Salvert, D. and Jouvet, M. (1979). Spinal projections from the lower brain stem in the cat demonstrated by the horseradish peroxidase technique. II — Projection from the dorsolateral pontine tegmentum and raphé nuclei. *Brain Res.,* **176**, 215–231.

Tricklebank, M. D., Hutson P. H. and Curzon G. (1982). Analgesia induced by brief foot-shock is inhibited by 5-hydroxytryptamine but unaffected by antagonists of 5-hydroxytryptamine or naloxone. *Neuropharmacol.,* **21**. 51–56.

Trousseau, A. and Pidoux, M. (1851). Electricité. Acupuncture. Electroacupuncture. In *Traité de thérapeutique et de matière médicale*. Vol. 1, Béchet Jeune, pp. 742–823.

Tyce, G. and Yaksh, T. (1981). Monoamine release from cat spinal cord by somatic stimuli: an intrinsic modulatory system. *J. Physiol.* (*Lond.*), **314**, 513–529.

Villanueva, L., Cadden, S. W., Chitour, D. and Le Bars, D. (1982). Diffuse Noxious Inhibitory Controls (DNIC): effects on glutamate-induced firing of dorsal horn neurones in the rat. *Neurosci. Lett.* (suppl.), **10**, *S507*.

Wagman, I. H. and Price, D. D. (1969). Responses of dorsal horn cells of M. mulatta to cutaneous and sural nerve A and C-fiber stimulation. *J. Neurophysiol.,* **32**, 803–817.

Wall, P. D. (1967). The laminar organization of dorsal horn and effects of escending impulses. *J. Physiol.* (*Lond.*), **188**, 403–423.

Wall, P. D. (1978). The gate control of pain mechanisms: a re-examination and re-statement. *Brain,* **101**, 1–18.

Wall, P. D. (1980). The substantia gelatinosa. A gate control mechanisms set across a sensory pathway. *Trends in Neurosciences,* **9**, 221–224.

Wall, P. D. and Sweet, W. H. (1967). Temporary abolition of pain in man. *Science,* **155**, 108–109.

Wand-Tetley, J. I. (1956). Historical methods of counter-irritation. *Ann. phys. Med.,* **3**, 90–98.

Wang, J. K. (1977). Antinociceptive effect of intrathecally administered serotonin. *Anesthesiology,* **47**, 269–271.

Watkins, L. R., Griffin, G., Leichnetz, G. I. R. and Mayer, D. J. (1980). The somatic organization of the nucleus raphé magnus and surrounding brain stem structures are revealed by HRP slow release gels. *Brain Res.,* **181**, 1–15.

Watkins, L. R., Cobelli, D. A., Faris, P., Aceto, M. D. and Mayer, D. J. (1982a). Opiate vs non-opiate footshock-induced analgsia (FSIA): the body region shocked is a critical factor. *Brain Res.,* **242**, 299–308.

Watkins, L. R. and Mayer, D. J. (1982b). Involvement of spinal opioid systems in footshock-induced analgsia: antagonism by naloxone is possible only before induction of analgesia. *Brain Res.,* **242**, 309–316.

Weil-Fugazza, J., Godefroy, F., Chitour, D. and Le Bars, D. (1981). Synthèse de la sérotonine au niveau spinal chez le rat: modifications induites par stimulation somatique nociceptive associée ou non à l'administration de morphine. *C. R. Acad. Sci., Paris,* **293**, 89–92.

Whitehorn, D. and Burgess, P. R. (1973). Changes in polarization of central branches of myelinated mechano-receptors and nociceptor fibers during noxious and innocuous stimulation of the skin. *J. Neurophysiol.,* **36**, 226–237.

Willer, J. C. (1977). Comparative study of perceived pain and nociceptive flexion reflex in man. *Pain,* **3**, 69–80.

Willer, J. C. and Albe-Fessard, D. (1980). Electrophysiological evidence for a release of endogenous opiates in stress-induced "analgesia" in man. *Brain Res.,* **198**, 419–426.

Willis, D. W. and Coggeshall, R. E. (1978). *Sensory mechanisms of the spinal cord.* Plenum Press, New York and London.

Willis, W. D., Haber, L. H. and Martin, R. F. (1977). Inhibition of spinothalmic tract cells and interneurons by brain stem stimulation in the monkey. *J. Neurophysiol.,* **40**, 968–981.

Yaksh, T. L. and Wilson, P. R. (1979). Spinal serotonin terminal system mediates antinociception. *J. Pharmacol. Exp. Ther.,* **208**, 446–453.

Young, W. S. and Kuhar, M. J. (1980). Serotonin receptor localization in rat brain by light microscopic autoradiography. *Eur. J. Pharmacol.,* **62**, 237–239.

Zemlan, F. P. and Pfaff, D. W. (1979). Topographical organization in medullary reticulo-spinal systems as demonstrated by the horseradish peroxidase technique. *Brain Res.,* **174**, 161–166.

Zieglgansberger, W. and Herz, A. (1971). Changes of cutaneous receptive fields of spinocervical tract neurons and other dorsal neurons by microelectrophoretically administered amino-acid. *Exp. Brain Res.,* **13**, 111–126.

Zieglgansberger, W. and Puil, E. A. (1973). Actions of glutamic acid on spinal neurones. *Exp. Brain Res.,* **17**, 35–49.

Zimmermann, M. (1977). Encoding in dorsal horn interneurons receiving noxious and non noxious afferents. *J. Physiol* (*Paris*), **73**, 221–232.

Stress-induced Analgesia
Edited by M. D. Tricklebank and G. Curzon

CHAPTER 5

Opioid and non-opioid stress analgesia

J.W. LEWIS, G. W. TERMAN, L. R. NELSON and J. C. LIEBESKIND

It has become increasingly clear that intrinsic to the brain and spinal cord are neural systems whose normal function is the inhibition of pain. This chapter describes our work exploring the neurochemistry, neuroanatomy, and endocrinology of these analgesia systems and our attempts to define the environmental stimuli required for their activation.

Reynolds (1969) was the first to demonstrate that electrical stimulation of a portion of the medial brainstem, the periaqueductal grey matter, produced analgesia in the rat so profound as to permit surgery without anaesthesia. Subsequently, Mayer *et al.* (1971) and many others have confirmed and greatly extended this original observation. Stimulation-produced analgesia is as potent as moderate to high doses of morphine measured in a variety of standard analgesiometric tests (e.g. Mayer *et al.*, 1971; Giesler and Liebeskind, 1976; Dennis *et al.*, 1980). This analgesia appears to represent a true pain suppression and is not secondary to changes in other sensory or motor systems (Mayer *et al.*, 1971). In general, this descending or centrifugal pain suppressive system seems to originate in the medial diencephalon or periaqueductal grey to descend from there to the nucleus raphé magnus and hence to the cord via the dorsolateral funiculus (see Fields and Basbaum, 1979; Lewis *et al.*, 1982a; Watkins and Mayer, 1982). The ultimate locus of pain inhibition due to stimulating any of these areas appears to be the dorsal horn of the spinal cord. Here lie the first central nociceptive neurones, and it is these neurones whose activity is preferentially blocked by analgesic brain stimulation (e.g. Oliveras *et al.*, 1974).

Akil *et al.* (1972, 1976b) reported that administration of naloxone, the specific opiate antagonist, significantly reduced stimulation-produced analgesia in the rat. This finding suggested that analgesia results from the liberation of endogenous opiate-like substances, an hypothesis that gained considerable support with the discovery of the opioid peptides (e.g. Hughes *et al.*, 1975; Li and Chung, 1976). Several other lines of evidence also indicate a significant role for opioid peptides in pain inhibition. Stimulation-produced analgesia manifests tolerance with repeated administration and cross-tolerance with morphine (Mayer and Hayes, 1975). Opiate binding sites and opioid peptide-containing cell bodies or fibre terminals are found in brain areas supporting the analgesia, areas where it may also be elicited by microinjections of opioid peptides and opiate drugs (e.g. Mayer and Price, 1976; Hökfelt *et al.*, 1977; Rossier *et al.*, 1977b; Yaksh and Rudy, 1978; Watson *et al.*, 1979). Lesions in this descending system block both stimulation-produced and opiate analgesia (Basbaum *et al.*, 1977). Stimulation-produced analgesia and analgesic doses of morphine or opioid peptides have a similar excitatory electrophysiological action on cellular activity within this medial brainstem substrate (e.g. Oleson *et al.*, 1978; Urca and Liebeskind, 1979).

However, it is becoming clear that not all intrinsic mechanisms of pain inhibition rely on this opioid path; multiple mechanisms exist involving separate or partly separate neurochemical and anatomical substrates. For example, several groups have failed to show naloxone antagonism of stimulation-produced analgesia (e.g. Pert and Walter, 1976; Yaksh *et al.*, 1976). A possible explanation for this discrepancy is suggested by the work of Cannon *et al.* (1982) who found that neurochemically discrete mechanisms appear to exist within the midline periaqueductal grey. Stimulation within and below the ventral periaqueductal grey caused analgesia that was sensitive to naloxone blockade, whereas more dorsal stimulation caused analgesia that was unaffected by this drug. Thus, opioid and non-opioid forms of stimulation-produced analgesia seem to involve adjacent regions of the midbrain.

A great deal of recent effort has been devoted to the search for natural, physiological triggers of the brain's intrinsic analgesia systems. It has been shown that exposure to a variety of stressors in the rat elicits pain suppression lasting for at least several minutes, as measured by standard analgesiometric tests (e.g., Chance *et al.*, 1977; Chesher and Chan, 1977; Madden *et al.*, 1977; Amir and Amit, 1978; Bodnar *et al.*, 1978a; Hayes *et al.*, 1978a; Jackson *et al.*, 1979; Lewis *et al.*, 1980a; Watkins *et al.*, 1982a). Such findings suggested that although pain is an important warning signal, there are certain emergency or stress conditions, under which pain *suppression* may be yet more adaptive. Thus, stress may be an important natural input to the endogenous analgesia systems of the brain at times when feeling pain could disrupt approprate coping behaviours (Liebeskind *et al.*, 1976).

Akil *et al.* (1976a) and Hayes *et al.* (1976) were the first to report that exposure to stress causes potent analgesia in rats. These studies differed, however, in one very important regard: Akil *et al.* (1976a) found that naloxone antagonized stress analgesia suggesting opioid involvement; Hayes *et al.* (1976) found that it did not. Subsequently, other investigators demonstrated stress analgesia in response to a host of stressors, but the question of opioid involvement remained controversial. To demonstrate clearly a role for opioid peptides in stress analgesia, several criteria must be satisfied: stress analgesia should be blocked by the opiate antagonist drug, naloxone; it should develop tolerance with repeated administration; and it should show cross-tolerance with opiate analgesia. When these criteria were applied to stress analgesia, some investigators obtained evidence of opioid involvement (Chesher and Chan, 1977; Madden *et al.*, 1977; Amir and Amit, 1978), but others did not (Bodnar *et al.*, 1978c; Hayes *et al.*, 1978a; Chance and Rosecrans, 1979a; 1979b).

It was at this time that our studies of stress analgesia began. Because qualitatively and quantitatively different stressors had been used in previous studies to produce analgesia (e.g., different parameters of footshock, rotation, oscillation, cold water swims, restraint, conditioned fear), their interpretation was difficult. Our goal was to investigate the phenomenon of stress analgesia systematically and to clarify what role, if any, was played by the opioid peptides. To this end, a single stressor, inescapable footshock, was selected and the temporal parameters of its administration were varied. This procedure allowed precise experimental control over the stressful stimulus and avoided the problems introduced by using qualitatively different stressors. Finally, we chose to assess pain sensitivity using the tail-flick test (D'Amour and Smith, 1941) and defined analgsia as an increse in latency to respond to radiant heat. It should be noted, however, that a variety of pain sensitivity tests have been used in laboratory animals (e.g. hot-plate, tail-flick, formalin tests, etc.); and the analgesic potencies of various agents (e.g. morphine, stress) have been shown to vary with the analgesia test employed (e.g., Dennis and Melzack, 1979; Kelly *et al.*, 1982).

OPIOID AND NON-OPIOID MECHANISMS OF STRESS ANALGESIA

We found that a single stressor, inescapable footshock, of constant intensity can elicit qualitatively different analgesic responses depending upon the temporal parameters of its application (Lewis *et al.*, 1980a). Exposure to prolonged, intermittent footshock, consisting of 1 s pulses of 3 mA (reduced to 2.5 mA in subsequent work) 60 Hz sine waves delivered every 5 s for 30 min (also reduced in subsequent work to 20 min) causes analgesia that is blocked by naloxone (10 mg/kg) (Figure 5.1). In subsequent work, this form of stress analgesia has been found to be antagonized by doses of naloxone as low as 0.1 mg/kg (Lewis *et al.*, 1980c) indicating the specificity of this opioid effect. In contrast, brief, continuous footshock, consisting of the same intensity current applied for 3 min, causes a roughly equipotent analgesia that is unaffected by even high doses of naloxone (Figure 5.1).

These results suggest the existence of at least two forms of stress analgesia, one that is mediated by opioid peptides and another that is not. The naloxone-sensitive analgesic response to prolonged, intermittent footshock satisfies two other

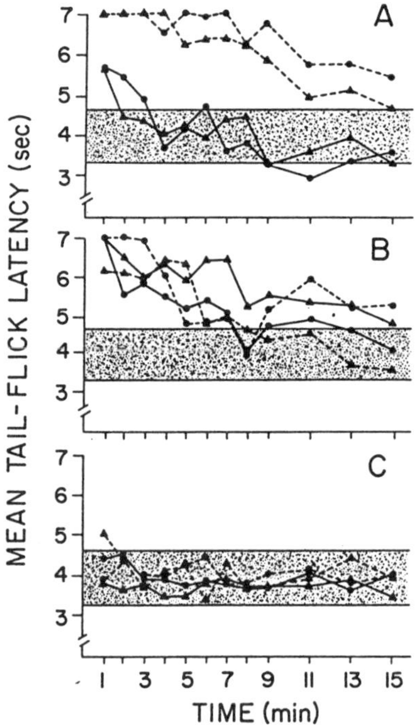

Figure 5.1 Mean tail-flick latencies of groups treated with naloxone (10 mg/kg, i.p., before and after shock; ●—●), naloxone vehicle (●- - -●), dexamethasone (0.4 mg/kg 24 h prior to and 0.2 mg/kg 2 h prior to test; ▲—▲), and dexamethasone vehicle (▲- - -▲) at 12 time periods beginning 1 min after exposure to (A) prolonged, intermittent footshock, (B) brief, continuous footshock, and (C) no footshock. The shaded areas represent ±2 standard errors of the grand mean calculated for the four non-stressed groups shown in (C). (Reprinted with permission, *Science,* **208**: 623–625, 1980.)

criteria for opioid involvement: It shows complete tolerance after 14 stress exposures (Lewis *et al.*, 1981c, Figure 5.2; see also Madden *et al.*, 1977) and is markedly reduced in morphine tolerant rats (Lewis *et al.*, 1981c; Figure 5.3). In contrast, brief stress analgesia appears independent of opioid mechanisms in

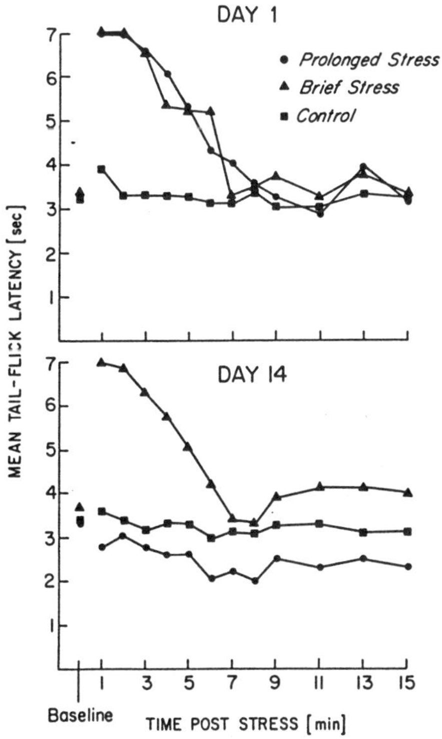

Figure 5.2 Development of tolerance to stress analgesia. Day 1: both prolonged and brief footshock stress elicited significantly elevated tail-flick latencies. Day 14: only the group repeatedly exposed to prolonged footshock developed tolerance to stress analgesia. (Reprinted with permission, *J. Neurosci.*, **1**: 358–363, 1981.)

that it shows no evidence of tolerance (Figure 5.2) or cross-tolerance with morphine (Lewis *et al.*, 1981c; Figure 5.3).

A further testament to the independence of these two forms of stress analgesia is the lack of development of cross-tolerance between them. Animals rendered tolerant to prolonged (opioid) footshock stress display normally robust analgesia in response to brief (non-opioid) footshock, and the analgesic response to prolonged footshock is still apparent in animals previously exposed to 14 brief stress sessions (Terman *et al.*, 1983a; Figure 5.4). These data also answer some questions regarding the mechanisms underlying tolerance to stress analgesia. It might have been suggested that tolerance to stress analgesia is due to sensory receptor adaptation, a central process of habituation, or to

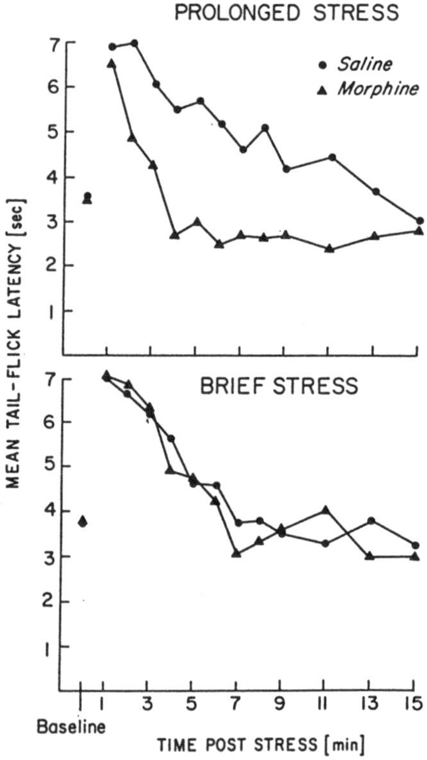

FIGURE 5.3 Effect of morphine tolerance on prolonged and brief footshock analgesia. Both footshock stressed elicited elevated tail-flick latencies in saline-treated control groups. Morphine tolerance significantly attenuated prolonged, but not brief, stress analgesia, indicating that only the form of stress analgesia sensitive to naloxone blockade (Figure 5.1) manifests cross-tolerance. (Reprinted with permission, *J. Neurosci.*, **1**: 358–363, 1981.)

non-specific changes (e.g. tissue damage to the paws). These explanations, however, seem unlikely. That an animal tolerant to the analgesic effect of prolonged footshock demonstrates normal analgesia to brief footshock argues against an explanation of tolerance based on peripheral receptor adaptation or tissue damage. Also, that repeated footshock caused diminution of only one form of stress analgesia suggests that this effect cannot be attributed to any general process such as habituation to stress. Thus, analgesic tolerance is not

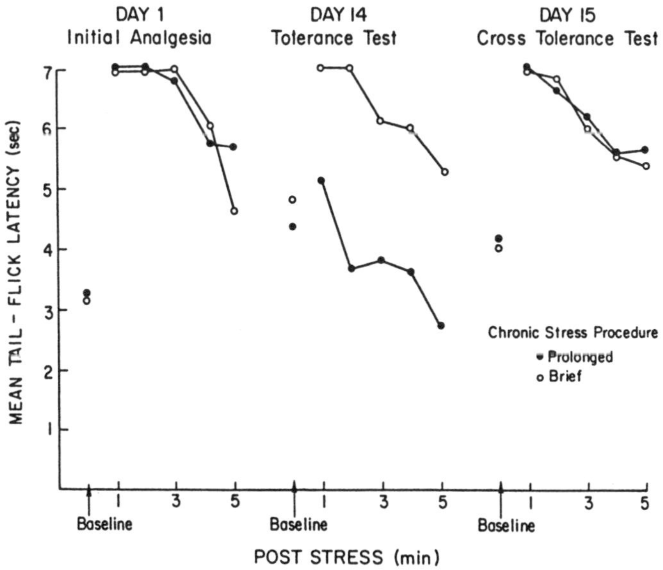

FIGURE 5.4 Lack of cross-tolerance between opioid and non-opioid stress analgesia. On Day 1, both stressors caused a potent analgesia. By Day 14, tolerance to the analgesic effect of prolonged (opioid), but not brief (non-opioid), footshock had developed. On Day 15, when rats received the footshock procedure that they had not yet experienced, the analgesic response to either stressor was as potent as that observed in naive rats on Day 1 indicating that cross-tolerance did not occur.

simply due to repetition of a stressor; rather the repeated stressor must be of a particular nature, opioid or non-opioid, for tolerance to occur.

Taken together, these results clearly indicate the existence of multiple endogenous analgesia systems that can be selectively accessed by different stressors. Moreover, the nature of the analgesia, opioid or non-opioid, elicited by stress appears dependent upon the temporal parameters of the stressful experience. The remainder of this chapter will be devoted to description of our work attempting to elucidate the hormonal, neurochemical, and neuroanatomical bases of these two forms of stress analgesia.

HORMONAL INFLUENCES IN STRESS ANALGESIA

The pituitary-adrenal and the sympatho-adrenal axes have long been recognized for their important roles in the adaptive response to stress (e.g. Selye, 1956). If pain suppression may be thought of as an adaptive response to certain stress conditions, participation of these hormonal systems in stress analgesia seems likely.

Several lines of evidence would suggest that pituitary hormones contribute importantly to the mediation of stress analgesia. First, the pituitary is a rich source of β-endorphin (Li and Chung, 1976), thought to be the most potent analgesic of the opioid peptides (Loh *et al.*, 1976). Stress has been shown to cause the release of pituitary opioids (Guillemin *et al.*, 1977; Rossier *et al.*, 1977a; Baizman *et al.*, 1979; Millan *et al.*, 1981; Akil *et al.*, 1982). Finally, stress analgesia (particularly those forms sensitive to naloxone blockade) is attenuated in hypophysectomized animals (Amir and Amit, 1979; Bodnar *et al*; Millan *et al.*, 1980; MacLennan *et al.*, 1982). Hypophysectomy, however, has been found ineffective in reducing some opioid forms of stress analgesia (Terman *et al.*, 1983b; Watkins *et al.*, 1982c) and most non-opioid forms (Chance *et al.*, 1979; Watkins *et al.*, 1982c). Consistent with such findings, we have reported (Lewis *et al.*, 1981b) that hypophysectomy reduces prolonged footshock (opioid) stress analgesia, but enhances brief (non-opioid) footshock analgesia (Figure 5.5).

Another peripheral source of opioid peptides is the adrenal medulla (e.g. Schultzberg *et al.*, 1978). The adrenal medulla contains enkephalin-like peptides that are stored and co-released with catecholamines (Viveros *et al.*, 1979; Livett *et al.*, 1981; for a recent review, see Viveros and Wilson, 1983) in response to sympathetic activation (e.g. Costa *et al.*, 1981) or trauma (Saria *et al.*, 1980). Although, the precise physiological function of these peptides remains to be determined, we have suggested that they are importantly involved in the analgesic response to certain forms of stress. Opioid, but not non-opioid, stress analgesia is markedly reduced by adrenalectomy, adrenal demedullation, or denervation of the adrenal medulla via coeliac ganglionectomy (Lewis *et al.*, 1982c; Figure 5.6). Because demedullation and ganglionectomy have as great an effect as removal of the entire adrenal gland, and because both basal and stressed adrenocortical function was unimpaired in adrenal denervated animals yet these rats failed to manifest opioid stress analgesia, we conclude that this form of stress analgesia depends specifically upon adrenal medullary, not cortical, function. Moreover, enkephalin-like peptides but not catecholamines, appear to be in its mediation. A dose of reserpine known to increase the adrenal content of enkephalins and their stimulation-induced release (Viveros *et al.*, 1980; Wilson *et al.*, 1980) significantly augments opioid stress analgesia (Lewis *et al.*, 1982c; Figure 5.7). This increased analgesia appears to reflect increased release of enkephalin-like peptides by stress rather than a non-specific drug effect in that the analgesia is still virtually eliminated by an opiate antagonist drug (Figure 5.7).

These behavioural observations have now been supported by recent biochemical evidence we have obtained in a collaborative study with Dr O. H. Viveros. Adrenal medullae were obtained from: (a) rats sacrificed immediately after exposure to either prolonged, brief, or no footshock stress; (b) rats subjected to chronic prolonged footshock stress (daily for 14 days) and

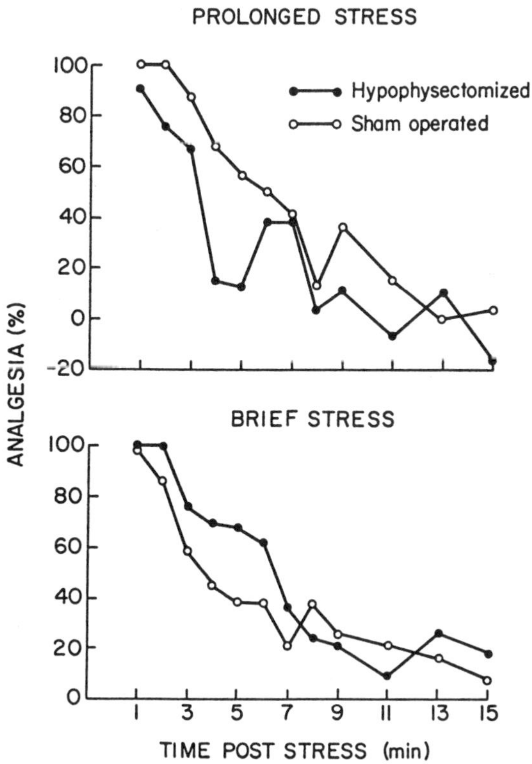

Figure 5.5 Mean degree of analgesia scores (per cent analgesia) following footshock stress. Hypophysectomy differentially affected stress analgesia: analgesia following prolonged stress was diminished, whereas that following brief stress was enhanced. (Reprinted with permission, *Proc. West. Pharmacol. Soc.*, **24**: 323–326, 1981.)

sacrificed either immediately or 24 h after the last stress session; and (c) rats treated with reserpine (2 mg/kg) on two successive days and subjected to prolonged or no footshock prior to sacrifice. Opiate-like material in the adrenal medulla was measured using a receptor binding assay (Chang and Cuatrecasas; 1979), and catecholamine content was determined fluorometrically (Anton and Sayre, 1962). The amount of opiate-like material in the adrenal medulla was significantly reduced by prolonged, but not by brief, footshock. Medullary enkephalin content was dramatically increased in reserpine treated rats, and this new elevated content was also reduced by exposure to prolonged stress. Finally, rats made tolerant to prolonged footshock analgsia (see Figure 5.2) no longer showed a depletion of adrenal enkephalin-like peptides after stress (Lewis *et al.*, 1982b; Table 5.1). These

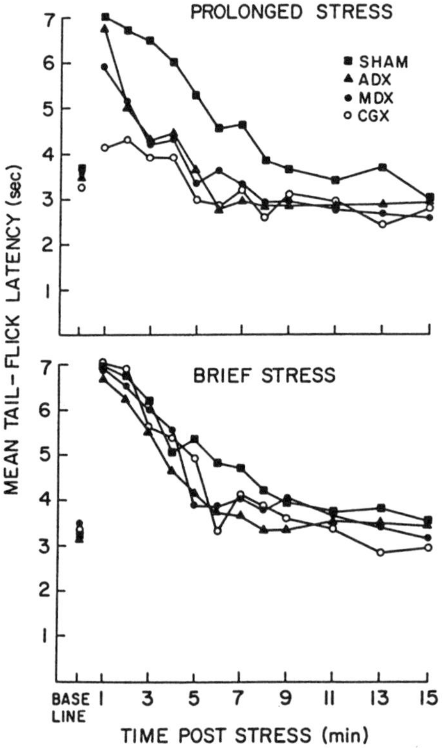

Figure 5.6 The effects of adrenalectomy (ADX), adrenal demedullation (MDX), denervation of the adrenal medulla by coeliac ganglionectomy (CGX), or sham surgery on the analgesic response to prolonged (opioid) and brief (non-opioid) footshock stress. ADX, MDX, and CGX all significantly attenuated opioid, but not non-opioid stress analgesia compared to shams. (Reprinted with permission, *Science,* **217**: 557–559, 1982.)

several converging lines of evidence strongly implicate adrenal enkephalin-like peptides in opioid stress analgesia. Several important questions, however, such as the locus of the opiate receptor mediating this analgesia (e.g. in the central nervous system or in the periphery), remain to be answered before this hypothesis can be fully accepted.

NEUROCHEMISTRY OF STRESS ANALGESIA

That hormonal opioid peptides appear critical for some forms of stress analgesia in no way precludes the involvement of central opioids as well. In

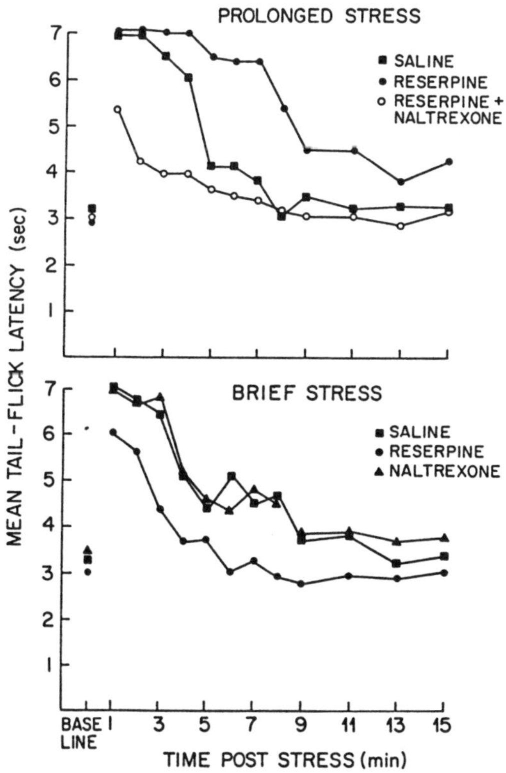

FIGURE 5.7 The effects of reserpine and naltrexone on the analgesic response to prolonged (opioid) and brief (non-opioid) footshock stress. Reserpine treatment significantly enhanced the analgesic response to prolonged stress. Even in the presence of reserpine, however, naltrexone antagonized this analgesia. Brief stress analgesia was significantly attenuated by reserpine but was not affected by naltrexone. (Reprinted with permission, *Science,* **217**: 557–559, 1982.)

fact, there is considerable evidence to indicate that stressors causing analgesia also alter one or another index of brain opioid activity (Akil *et al.*, 1976a; Madden *et al.*, 1977; Chance *et al.*, 1978; Rossier *et al.*, 1978; Lewis *et al.*, 1981a; Millan *et al.*, 1981). Undoubtedly, a number of other central neurotransmitter substances are involved in the mediation of opioid and non-opioid forms of stress analgesia. Our work has demonstrated an important role for acetylcholine in opioid stress analgesia (Lewis *et al.*, 1983a) and for histamine in non-opioid stress analgesia (Terman *et al.*, 1982a; 1982b). The reader is referred to other chapters in this volume by Bodnar and by Hutson *et*

Table 5.1 Effects of footshock stress on adrenal medullary opiate-like material and catecholamine content

Group	Opiate-like material (pmol/pair)	Total catecholamines (nmol/pair)
Control	0.70 ± 0.10	52.7 ± 3.0
Acute prolonged stress	0.42 ± 0.05*	54.3 ± 7.1
Acute brief stress	0.61 ± 0.09	61.9 ± 4.8
Reserpine	1.58 ± 0.24*	16.1 ± 2.6*
Reserpine + prolonged stress	1.23 ± 0.22*	17.3 ± 4.6*
Chronic prolonged stress, no stress prior to sacrifice	0.96 ± 0.12	54.5 ± 8.9
Chronic prolonged stress, stress prior to sacrifice	1.54 ± 0.29*	69.1 ± 8.1*

Values show means ± s.e.m.
*Differed from control (*t*-test, $p < 0.05$)

al. for descriptions of the importance of other neuropeptides and monoamines in stress analgesia.

Acetylcholine has long been thought to be involved in central mechanisms of anti-nociception. Cholinomimetic drugs can cause analgesia (see Pedigo and Dewey, 1981 for review); and when centrally administered, the brain loci most sensitive to these agents correspond well to those areas most sensitive to opiate microinjections and to electrical stimulation produced analgesia (Pert and Maxey, 1975; Mayer and Price, 1976). Anatomically, muscarinic cholinergic receptors are present in, among other places, portions of the midbrain and spinal cord involved in pain modulation (Wamsley *et al.*, 1981). We find that opioid, but not non-opioid, stress analgesia is reduced by scopolamine, a muscarinic cholinergic antagonist drug (Lewis *et al.*, 1983a; Figure 5.8). Antagonism of opioid stress analgesia by scopolamine was dose dependent with 0.1 mg/kg being the lowest effective dose. Importantly, methylscopolamine, a muscarinic cholinergic antagonist with only peripheral activity, failed to affect the analgesic response to prolonged footshock (Figure 5.8). That acetylcholine serves to stimulate the release of opioid peptides involved in pain inhibition, is suggested by the finding that oxotremorine, a potent muscarinic agonist, causes analgesia sensitive to opiate antagonist blockade (e.g. Howes *et al.*, 1969; Lewis *et al.*, 1983a; Pedigo and Dewey, 1981). We therefore conclude that a muscarinic cholinergic synapse exists in the central opioid pathway mediating stress analgesia.

Very little is known of the neurochemistry of non-opioid analgesia systems. Understanding of these systems may prove to be clinically relevant since if they

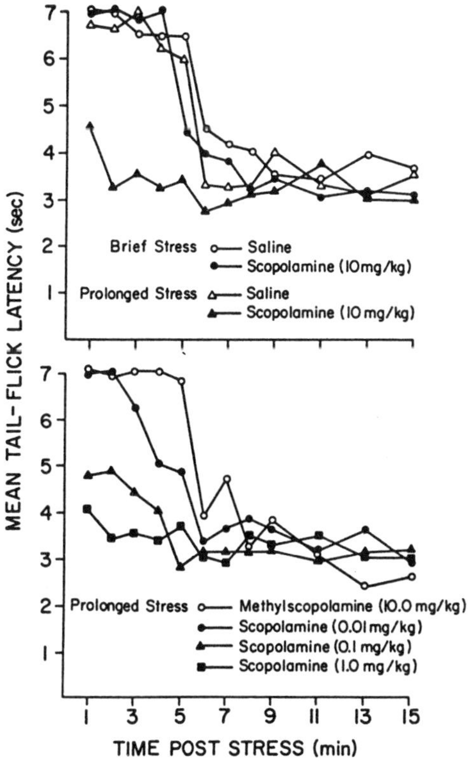

FIGURE 5.8 Effects of scopolamine on stress analgesia. *Top* — Prolonged and brief stress elicited a potent analgesia in saline-treated rats. Scopolamine (10 mg/kg) antagonized only prolonged stress analgesia. *Bottom* — Antagonism of prolonged stress analgesia by scopolamine was dose dependent. Significant reductions occurred at 1.0 and 0.1 but not 0.01 mg/kg. Methylscopolamine, a peripherally acting muscarinic cholinergic antagonist, was without effect. (Reprinted with permission, *Brain Res.*)

can be harnessed and utilized therapeutically, perhaps many of the problems associated with opioid analgesia (e.g. tolerance and dependence) could be avoided. Our studies of the pharmacology of non-opioid systems began with the observation that non-opioid stress analgesia was reduced by reserpine (Terman *et al.*, 1981; Lewis *et al.*, 1982c; Figure 5.7). Reserpine is a relatively non-specific drug in that it affects all monoaminergic neurones. Attempting to define which monoamine is critical, we were unable to attenuate non-opioid stress analgesia with specific dopamine, norepinephrine, or serotonin receptor antagonist or depletor drugs (e.g. haloperidol, propranolol, phentolamine, methysergide, α-methyl-*p*-tyrosine, *p*-chlorophenylalanine, disulfiram). In fact, this analgesia was enhanced by haloperidol. The monoaminergic agonist drugs, apomorphine, clonidine, and 5-methoxy-*N,N*-dimethyltryptamine, also did not reduce, but potentiated non-opioid stress analgesia (Terman *et al.*, 1982a; Table 5.2). Non-opioid stress analgesia, however, does appear to depend on the monoamine, histamine. This form of stress analgesia appears to rely specifically on the H_1 histamine receptor in that it is reduced by diphenhydramine, an H_1 receptor blocker, but not by cimetidine, an H_2 antagonist (Terman *et al.*, 1982a; Figure 5.9). Furthermore, it seems that histamine of neuronal origin is crucial as non-opioid stress analgesia is reduced by depletion of neuronal and mast cell histamine stores by α-fluoromethylhistidine, an inhibitor of histidine decarboxylase (required for histamine synthesis), but is unaffected by administration of Compound 48/80, which depletes histamine only from mast cells (Terman *et al.*, 1982b; Figure 5.10). That histamine is involved in central mechanisms of antinociception is supported by the demonstration of histamine in brain regions thought to be involved in

Table 5.2 Effects of monoamine drugs on brief (3 min) footshock stress analgesia

		Time post-stress (min)		
Drug	N	1–4	5–8	9–12
Depleting agents				
Reserpine (2 mg/kg)	14	4.44*	3.40*	2.92
p-Chlorophenylalanine and α-methyl-*p*-tyrosine	8	6.44	4.83	4.50
p-Chlorophenylalanine (300 mg/kg)	8	6.59	5.36	4.37
α-Methyl-*p*-tyrosine (250 mg/kg)	8	6.51	5.27	4.03
Disulfiram (150 mg/kg)	8	6.74	4.57	2.86
Receptor antagonists				
Haloperidol (0.2 mg/kg)	8	7.00	5.44*	4.38*
Methysergide (2 mg/kg)	8	6.94	4.94	3.93
Propranolol (5 mg/kg)	8	6.94	5.01	3.04
Phentolamine (10 mg/kg)	10	6.56	4.29	2.80
Diphenhydramine (25 mg/kg)	14	4.82*	3.45*	3.00
Receptor agonists				
Apomorphine (1 mg/kg)	10	6.70	6.56*	4.22*
5-Methoxy-*N,N*-dimethyltryptamine (2 mg/kg)	10	6.93	5.99*	4.54*
Clonidine (0.1 mg/kg)	10	7.00	5.72*	4.29*
Vehicle	92	6.73	4.68	3.21

See Terman *et al.*, (1982) for further details regarding drug administration procedures.
*Significantly different from appropriate vehicle control ($p < 0.05$)
Data displayed represent mean tail-flick latencies (s).

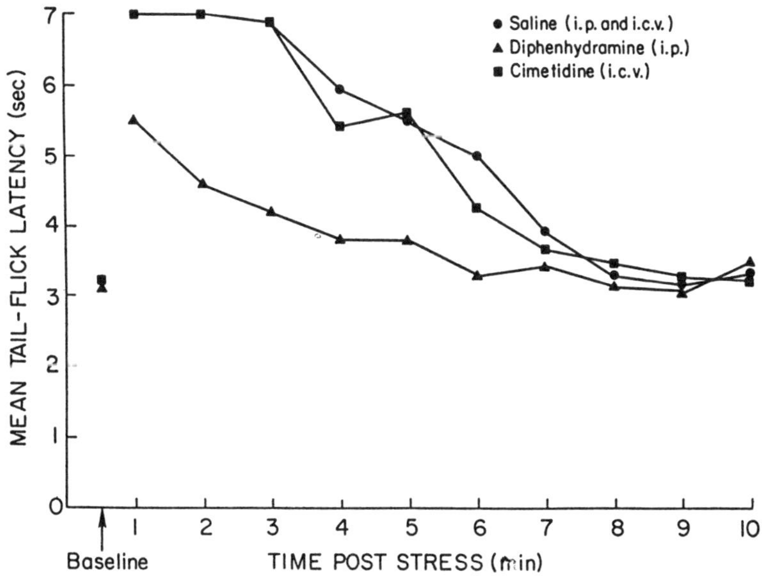

FIGURE 5.9 Non-opioid stress analgesia is significantly reduced by the histamine H_1 receptor antagonist drug, diphenhydramine (25 mg/kg, i.p.), but not by the H_2 antagonist, cimetidine (50 μg/rat, i.c.v.).

pain-inhibition (see Schwartz *et al.*, 1981) and by the fact that analgesia follows microinjections of histamine into these areas (Glick and Crane, 1978).

NEUROANATOMY OF STRESS ANALGESIA

As already described, endogenous pain-inhibitory systems acted upon by opiate drugs and activated by electrical stimulation originate within the brain stem, involve areas such as the periaqueductal grey matter and nucleus raphé magnus, and function by exerting descending or centrifugal control over the responsiveness of nociceptive neurones in the dorsal horn of the spinal cord. The neuroanatomical substrates of opioid and non-opioid stress analgesia appear to overlap considerably with these brain and spinal systems.

Spinal pathways, particularly the dorsolateral funiculus, have been implicated in stimulation-produced and opiate analgesia (e.g. Basbaum *et al.*, 1977) and, more recently, in footshock induced analgesia (Hayes *et al.*, 1978b; Chance, 1980; Watkins *et al.*, 1982b). We find that the analgesic responses to prolonged intermittent, and brief continuous, footshock rely to some extent on the integrity of the dorsolateral funiculus (Lewis *et al.*, 1983b; Figure 5.11). Thus, opioid and non-opioid stress analgesia share a common substrate, the dorsolateral funiculus, and both rely on descending neural influences.

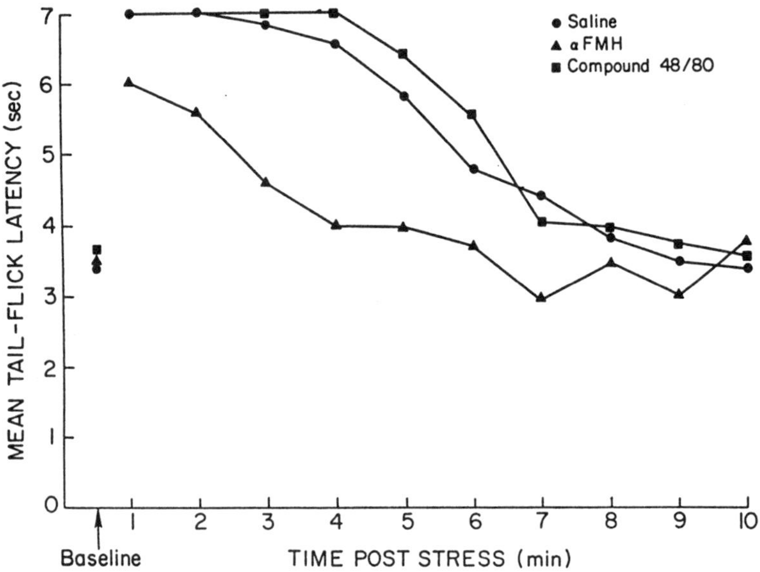

Figure 5.10 Administration of α-fluoromethylhistidine (100 mg/kg, i.p.) causes a depletion of neuronal and mast cell stores of histamine by inhibition of its synthetitic enzyme, histidine decarboxylase, and a concomitant reduction in non-opioid stress analgesia. This form of stress analgesia appears to rely specifically on histamine of neuronal origin in that it was not affected by depletion of only mast cell histamine by Compound 48/80 (2mg/kg, i.p., daily for 2 days).

A possible source of dorsolateral funiculus fibres critical to stress analgesia is the nucleus raphé magnus, a cell group whose axons project to the spinal cord via this path (see Fields and Basbaum, 1979; Watkins *et al.*, 1980). That this nucleus is involved in endogenous mechanisms of anti-nociception is suggested by findings such as the following: its electrical stimulation causes analgesia (e.g. Oliveras *et al.*, 1977; Fields and Basbaum, 1979); it is sensitive to microinjection of opiates (e.g. Azami *et al.*, 1982); and lesioning it blocks stimulation-provoked analgesia derived from more rostral sites (Prieto *et al.*, 1983). Association of the nucleus raphé magnus specifically with either opioid or non-opioid analgesia systems, however, is difficult. Some workers report the analgesia produced by stimulating it is reduced by naloxone (Oliveras *et al.*, 1977; Zorman *et al.*, 1981), whereas others disagree (Satoh *et al.*, 1980). In our work, complete electrolytic lesions of the raphé magnus (destroying 85% of the nucleus; Figure 5.12) reduced the non-opioid form of stress analgesia but did not affect the opioid form (Cannon *et al.*, 1983; Figure 5.13). These lesions, consistent with previous reports of others (e.g. Azami *et al.*, 1982), attenuate the analgesic effects of systemically adminis-

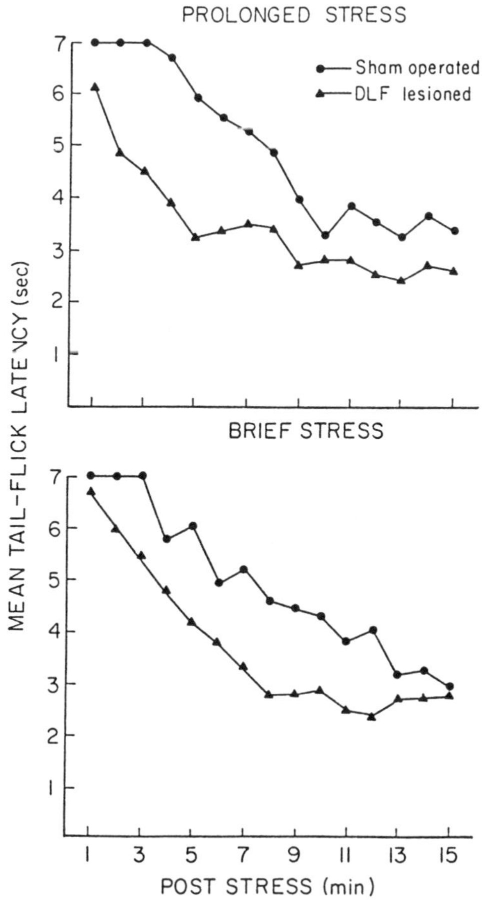

Figure 5.11 Lesions of the spinal dorsolateral funiculus, at either C3 or T2 (data combined as DLF lesioned), significantly reduced prolonged and brief footshock stress analgesia. (Reprinted with permission, *Brain Res.*)

tered morphine. This latter result suggests that although morphine and opioid stress analgesia have been shown to be similar in many respects (e.g. antagonism by naloxone, tolerance, and cross-tolerance), their anatomical substrates are not entirely identical.

Yet another indication that stress can activate central nervous system pain-inhibitory pathways derives from the finding that cross-tolerance develops between opioid stress analgesia and opioid mediated stimulation-produced analgesia (Penner *et al.*, 1982). Rats were implanted with two

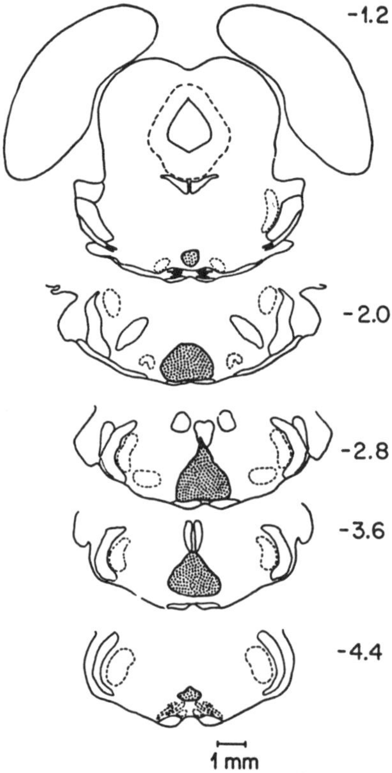

Figure 5.12 A representative lesion extending from the medial n. of the trapezoid body to the inferior olive and destroying greater than 95% of the nucleus raphé magnus. (Drawings were adapted from the atlas of Pelligrino *et al.* Reprinted with permission, *Brain Res.*)

electrodes in the periaqueductal grey matter. Stimulating the dorsal electrode caused analgesia which was insensitive to naloxone blockade, whereas stimulating the ventral electrode caused naloxone sensitive analgesia (see also, Cannon *et al.*, 1982). Stimulation thresholds for both types of analgesia were determined in each animal before and after exposure to 14 days of either prolonged intermittent (opioid) or brief continuous (non-opioid) footshock stress. Opioid stress led to tolerance to the analgesic effects of stress and elevated thresholds for elicitation of analgesia by ventral stimulation. However, thresholds for elicitation of analgesia by dorsal stimulation were unaffected and neither threshold was affected by prior exposure to the non-opioid stress.

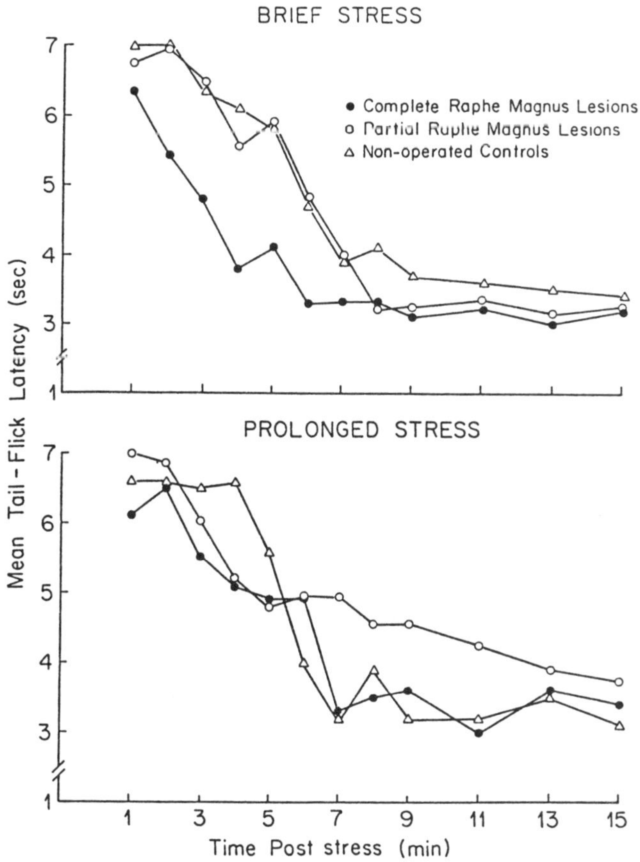

FIGURE 5.13 Complete, but not partial, raphé magnus lesions significantly attenuated the analgesic response to brief footshock. The analgesia following prolonged footshock was unaffected by these lesions. (Reprinted with permission, *Brain Res.*)

EARLY EXPERIENCE INFLUENCES STRESS ANALGESIA

An ample literature suggests that administration of adrenal corticosteroids or simply handling animals during the perinatal period can profoundly influence the behavioural and endocrinological response to stress in adulthood (for review, see Ader, 1975). How these perinatal manipulations specifically affect the adult analgesic response to stress is unknown, although neonatally administered stress can alter brain enkephalin levels (Torda, 1978) and affect the analgesic responsiveness to morphine (Bardo *et al.*, 1981). Moreover, Bodnar and co-workers demonstrated that certain perinatal pharmacological treatments influence some forms of stress analgesia. Thus neonatal administration of monosodium glutamate in rats, which causes destruction of β-endorphin-containing neurones in the hypothalamic arcuate nucleus, attenuates the analgesia caused by exposure to cold water swim in adulthood (Bodnar *et al.*, 1978a, 1980).

Prenatal exposure to ethanol can markedly influence later sensitivity to stress. When tested as adults, rats exposed to ethanol *in utero* exhibit a potentiated corticosterone response to certain stressors (cardiac puncture or noise and shake), but not to others (fasting or cold stress) (Taylor *et al.*, 1982). We now find that prenatal ethanol exposure can interfere specifically with the analgesic response to opioid mediated stress in the adult rat (Nelson *et al.*, 1982). Female rats prenatally exposed to ethanol were tested at approximately 150 days of age for their analgesic response to prolonged, intermittent (2.5 mA, 1s on per 5s for 10min) and brief, continuous (2.5 mA, on for 2min) footshock. These two sets of footshock parameters elicited naloxone-sensitive (opioid) and naloxone-insensitive (non-opioid) forms of stress analgesia, respectively. Compared to controls, rats with foetal ethanol exposure showed a markedly potentiated opioid stress analgesia (Nelson *et al.*, 1982). Non-opioid stress analgesia was unaffected. These results add prolonged, intermittent footshock to the list of stressors to which rats prenatally exposed to ethanol are more sensitive and suggest that this prenatal experience produces long-term effects on the functioning of endogenous opioid analgesia systems.

EVIDENCE FOR TWO INDEPENDENT OPIOID FORMS OF STRESS ANALGESIA

Recently, we have found (Terman *et al.*, 1983b) that 3min of continuous footshock (2.5 mA; 60Hz) which we have previously seen to elicit non-opioid stress analgesia (Lewis *et al.*, 1981c), can in some animals provoke stress analgesia sensitive to naltrexone antagonism. By systematically varying duration of exposure while holding other footshock parameters constant, we have now established that 3min is intermediate between those durations eliciting clearly opioid and clearly non-opioid stress analgesias. Thus, robust naltrexone antagonism of continuous footshock stress analgesia was observed at 1 and 2min footshock durations, whereas a comparable degree of analgesia elicited by the same footshock but applied continuously for 4 or 5min was completely insensitive to this drug. Further characterization of these forms of stress analgesia revealed that the analgesic response to 1min of continuous footshock develops tolerance after 14 exposures, and manifests cross-tolerance both with morphine and with the prolonged (20min) intermittent (opioid) form of stress analgesia described previously. The analgesic response to 4min of continuous footshock, by contrast, does not develop tolerance, is unaffected by morphine tolerance, is not cross-tolerant with either the 1 min continuous or 20 min intermittent forms of opioid stress analgesia, and hence presumably is mediated by non-opioid mechanisms (Terman *et al.*, 1983b).

These findings reinforce our previous contention that exposure to brief continuous footshock can cause a non-opioid form of stress analgesia. It is now clear that 4 or 5 min of this stress provide a more purely non-opioid type of stress analgesia than the 3 min used in our earlier studies. Moreover, a still briefer exposure to continuous footshock (1 or 2 min) was seen to induce a clearly opioid form of stress analgesia according to several standard criteria of opioid involvement. It then became of interest to compare the two opioid forms. Therefore, several studies were conducted (Terman *et al.*, 1983b) comparing the 1 min continuous and 20 min intermittent footshock parameters. We find that both are sensitively antagonized by naloxone (0.1 mg/kg), both develop tolerance and cross-tolerance with morphine, and each manifests cross-tolerance with the other. In fact, both show cross-tolerance with the naloxone-sensitive form of stimulation-produced analgesia (Cannon *et al.*, 1982; Penner *et al.*, 1982). However, these two clearly opioid forms of stress analgesia are also quite different in certain respects. Whereas, the analgesic response to the 20 min intermittent footshock is reduced by hypophysectomy (Lewis *et al.*, 1981b), is dependent upon adrenal medullary enkephalin-like peptides (Lewis *et al.*, 1982c), and relies on central muscarinic cholinergic mechanisms (Lewis *et al.*, 1983a), the analgesia following 1 min of continuous footshock is independent of these hormonal and cholinergic systems and hence presumably dependent on opioids of central, but not peripheral, origin (Terman *et al.*, 1983b).

In further work we have found that the opioid or non-opioid nature of the analgesic effect of continuous footshock depends not only on duration of exposure (1 min versus 4 min), but also on current intensity. For example, 3 min of continuous footshock at 1.5 or 2.0 mA elicits a naltrexone blockable analgesia, whereas 3 min of a more intense shock (3.0 or 3.5 mA) causes analgesia insensitive to naltrexone blockade. Considering either the intensity or duration of continuous footshock parameters, therefore, it appears that the values used in our earlier work (2.5 mA for 3 min) are slightly higher than optimal for eliciting opioid stress analgesia and slightly lower than optimal for eliciting stress analgesia of the non-opioid sort. It is important to add, however, that whereas small increments in continuous footshock stress cause a sudden shift from an opioid to a non-opioid mechanism, application of exactly the same total amount of footshock as that yielding non-opioid analgesia, but applying it intermittently rather than continuously, once again evokes an opioid form (although a different opioid form) of stress analgesia.

Interestingly, continuous footshock (2.5 mA for 1 or 4 min) can elicit analgesia in rats given a surgical level of anaesthesia with pentobarbital (55 mg/kg) (Terman *et al.*, 1983b). Stress analgesia in these animals, measured by the tail-flick test, is indistinguishable from that displayed by unanaesthetized controls in either magnitude, duration, or sensitivity to naltrexone. On the other hand, the analgesic response to 20 min of intermittent footshock is completely abolished by anaesthesia (Terman *et al.*, 1983b; see also, Jensen and Smith, 1981). This finding provides another difference between the two opioid forms of stress analgesia elicited by continuous versus intermittent footshock. It also reveals that some forms of stress analgesia can be studied under surgical anaesthesia with resultant practical or ethical advantage but other forms, unfortunately, cannot.

SUMMARY AND CONCLUSIONS

These studies provide compelling evidence that exposure to stress is an adequate stimulus for the activation of endogenous pain-inhibitory mechanisms. Moreover, our findings indicate that stress analgesia is not a unitary phenomenon. Multiple, neurochemically, neuroanatomically, and hormonally different analgesia substrates appear to exist. Which of these is called into play appears to depend on remarkably slight variations in the temporal or intensive properties of the footshock stress stimulus. Our initial results (Lewis *et al.*, 1980a) provided the first unequivocal demonstration that a single stressor, inescapable footshock, can selectively activate either an opioid or a non-opioid mediated endogenous analgesia system.

The analgesic response to 20 min of intermittent footshock appears to be mediated by opioid peptides (Lewis *et al.*, 1980a, 1981c). It depends upon hormonal factors, particularly enkephalin-like peptides of the adrenal medulla (Lewis *et al.*, 1981b, 1982b, 1982c). It involves central muscarinic cholinergic mechanisms (Lewis *et al.*, 1983a) and depends on the integrity of a descending spinal pathway, the dorsolateral funiculus (Lewis *et al.*, 1983b).

By contrast, the analgesic response to brief (3 min) continuous footshock appears to be non-opioid (Lewis *et al.*, 1980a, 1981c). It relies on the nucleus raphé magnus (Cannon *et al.*, 1983) and the dorsolateral funiculus (Lewis *et al.*, 1983b), and the putative neurotransmitter, histamine, may be importantly involved in its mediation (Terman *et al.*, 1982a; 1982b).

Recently, we have described another opioid form of stress analgesia elicited by exposure to 1 or 2 min of continuous footshock. It is similar to that caused by 20 min of intermittent footshock in that it is blocked by opiate antagonists, develops tolerance, and shows cross-tolerance with morphine and with the stress analgesia caused by 20 min intermittent shock. However, these two opioid forms of stress analgesia are not the same. The one provoked by 20 min of intermittent footshock, but not the one resulting from 1 min of continuous footshock, is dependent on the integrity of the pituitary and adrenal medulla and is eliminated by barbiturate anaesthesia.

During the course of our research, work from two other laboratories has contributed significantly to an understanding of selective activation of opioid and non-opioid analgesia systems by stress. Watkins and her colleagues reported that opioid or non-opioid stress analgesia can be elicited depending upon the region of the body receiving noxious stimulation. Footshock restricted to the forepaws causes analgesia that is antagnized by naloxone and cross-tolerant with morphine analgesia. Footshock given to only the hindpaws or to all four paws causes analgesia that is non-opioid (see Watkins and Mayer, 1982). Furthermore, the type of stress analgesia described by Watkins is similar to the type we have studied in that both opioid and non-opioid forms rely on the dorsolateral funiculus (Lewis *et al.*, 1983b; Watkins *et al.*, 1982b) and lesions of the nucleus raphé magnus block the non-opioid form (Cannon *et al.*, 1983; Watkins *et al.*, 1981). Her results differ from ours, however, primarily in that forepaw shock (opioid) analgesia is not dependent on the integrity of the pituitary or adrenal medulla (Lewis *et al.*, 1982c; Watkins *et al.*, 1982c). It appears that the opioid stress analgesia she has studied is more related to the 1 min continuous footshock form of opioid stress analgesia we have recently revealed.

Work from Maier's laboratory has shown that elicitation of opioid and non-opioid forms of analgesia can depend upon the ability of the subject to control the stressful situation. In their initial work, groups of rats were given an equivalent amount of either escapable or inescapable tail-shocks. Twenty-four hours later, in response to a reminder shock, those rats receiving inescapable, but not those receiving escapable, tail-shock displayed a pronounced analgesia (Jackson *et al.*, 1979) mediated by opioid peptides (Maier *et al.*, 1980). Subsequently, they found that the analgesia reinstated 24 h after 80 inescapable tail-shocks is cross-tolerant with morphine analgesia (Drugan *et al.*, 1981), and is blocked by dexamethasone, hypophysectomy, and adrenalectomy (MacLennan *et al.*, 1982). If pain sensitivity is assessed immediately after the tail-shock procedure, 80 inescapable tail-shocks cause analgesia that is blocked by naltrexone, whereas 20 tail-shocks cause an equipotent analgesia insensitive to this drug (Grau *et al.*, 1981). These findings parallel ours in a number of ways:

(1) Analgesias due to inescapable and prolonged footshock are both cross-tolerant with morphine and blocked by naloxone, dexamethasone, hypophysectomy, and adrenalectomy;
(2) Twenty inescapable shocks produce a naloxone-insensitive analgesia and 80 inescapable shocks produce a naloxone-sensitive analgesia (analogous to the effects of brief and prolonged footshock respectively);
(3) Both procedures that elicit opioid dependent stress analgesia (prolonged, intermittent footshock and 60–80 tail-shocks), but not those causing non-opioid dependent stress analgesia (3 min continuous footshock and

20–40 tail-shocks), produce learned helplessness as assessed by a shuttlebox escape task and analgesia that can be reinstated by a reminder shock 24 h later (Maier *et al.*, 1983).

One difference, however, is that the opioid analgesia described by Maier's group depends on the adrenal cortex (MacLennan *et al.*, 1982), whereas the opioid analgesia we have described depends on the adrenal medulla (Lewis *et al.*, 1982c). This apparent discrepancy may perhaps be accounted for by the fact that we measured the analgesic response immediately following stress, whereas MacLennan *et al.* derive from studies of analgesia reinstated 24 h after stress.

Studies of stress analgesia may ultimately prove to be of both practical and theoretical value. Stress analgesia seems to provde a useful tool for studying environmental activation of endogenous analgesia systems and for investigating their neurochemistry. Although production of analgesia by exposure to stress is obviously not clinically applicable, investigating this phenomenon may lead to a better understanding of therapeutic techniques such as acupuncture and placebo analgesia, which are suspected of being opioid mediated (e.g., Mayer *et al.*, 1976; Pomeranz and Chiu, 1976; Levine *et al.*, 1978) and hypnotic analgesia, which is thought to be non-opioid in nature (Goldstein and Hilgard, 1975; Mayer *et al.*, 1976). Clearly, we still know very little about the conditions under which endogenous pain-inhibitory systems are active and what natural stimuli or environmental circumstances call them into play. There is some evidence to suggest that opioids are released tonically (Jacob *et al.*, 1974; Berntson and Walker, 1977), at least during certain hours of the day (Frederickson *et al.*, 1977), and serve to modulate pain sensitivity; but it is widely held to be the case that such tonic release is at best slight and that opioids active in pain suppression are released principally in a phasic manner, triggered by specific internal or external events (see Lewis *et al.*, 1980b; Sherman and Liebeskind, 1980). Our work, and that of others, may prove heuristic in suggesting conditions under which stress is an adequate stimulus for activating either opioid or non-opioid mechanisms of pain inhibition. Although, at best, inescapable footshock merely models natural stress conditions, it is proving useful as a highly precise, reliable, and controllable probe for elucidating anatomical substrates and neurochemical mechanisms of anti-nociception. As we have seen, even very small variations in footshock parameters can strikingly shift the neurochemical foundation of stress analgesia from dependence on to independence of opioid peptides. More naturalistic work by others, suggesting that sexual behaviour (Crowley *et al.*, 1977), fighting (Miczek *et al.*, 1982), and food deprivation (Bodnar *et al.*, 1978b; McGivern *et al.* 1979, 1980) can be adequate stimuli for triggering opioid or non-opioid analgesia systems apparently similar to those we are studying, encourages the belief that a *rapprochement* between these more mechanistic and naturalistic kind of studies can ultimately be made.

ACKNOWLEDGEMENTS

The authors wish to express particular thanks to Drs J. Timothy Cannon and Jack E. Sherman for their valuable contributions to this research. Our work is supported by NIH grant NS07628 and a gift from the Brotman Foundation.

REFERENCES

Ader, R. (1975). Early experience and hormones: emotional behavior and adrenocortical function, in *Hormonal Correlates of Behavior* (eds B. E. Eleftheriou and R. Sprott), pp. 7–33, Plenum Press, New York.

Akil, H., Mayer, D. J., and Liebeskind, J. C. (1972). Comparaison chez le rat entre l'analgesie par stimulation de la substance grise peri-aqueducale et l'analgesie morphinique, *C.R. Acad. Sci. (Paris)*, **274**, 3603–3605.

Akil, H., Madden, J., Patrick, R. L., and Barchas, J. D. (1976a). Stress-induced increase in endogenous opiate peptides; concurrent analgesia and its partial reversal by naloxone, in *Opiates and Endogenous Opioid Peptides* (ed. H. W. Kosterlitz), pp. 63–70, Elsevier, Amsterdam.

Akil, H., Mayer, D. J., and Liebeskind, J. C. (1976b). Antagonism of stimulation-produced analgesia by naloxone, a narcotic antagonist. *Science,* **191**, 961–962.

Akil, H., Ueda, Y., Lin, H-L., Lewis, J. W., Walker, J. M., Shiomi, H., Liebeskind, J. C., and Watson, S. J. (1981). Multiple forms of beta-endorphin in pituitary and brain: effect of stress, in *Advances in Endgoneous and Exogenous Opioid Peptides* (eds H. Takagi and E. Simon), pp. 116–118, Kodansha Press, Tokyo.

Amir, S., and Amit, Z. (1978). Endogenous opioid ligands may mediate stress-induced changes in the affective properties of pain related behavior in rats. *Life Sci.,* **23**, 1143–1152.

Amir, S., and Amit, Z. (1979). The pituitary gland mediates acute and chronic pain responsiveness in stressed and non-stressed rats. *Life Sci.,* **24**, 439–448.

Anton, A. H., and Sayre, D. F. (1962). A study of the factors affecting the aluminium oxide-trihydroxyindole procedure for the analysis of catecholamines. *J. Pharmacol. exp. Ther.,* **138**, 360–375.

Azami, J., Llewelyn, M. B., and Roberts, H. H. T. (1982). The contribution of nucleus reticularis paragigantocellularis and nucleus raphé magnus to the analgesia produced by systemically administered morphine, investigated with the microinjection technique. *Pain,* **12**, 229–246.

Baizman, E. R., Cox, B. M., Osman, O. H., and Goldstein, A. (1979). Experimental alterations of endorphin levels in rat pituitary. *Neuroendocrinology,* **28**, 402–424.

Bardo, M. T., Bhatnagar, R. K., and Gebhart, G. F. (1981). Opiate receptor ontogeny and morphine-induced effects: influence of chronic footshock stress in preweanling rats. *Dev. Brain Res.,* **1**, 487–495.

Basbaum, A. I., Marley, N. J., O'Keefe, J., and Clanton, C. H. (1977). Reversal of morphine and stimulus produced analgesia by subtotal spinal cord lesions. *Pain,* **3**, 43–56.

Berntson, G. G., and Walker, J. M. (1977). Effect of opiate receptor blockade on pain sensitivity in the rat. *Brain Res. Bull.,* **2**, 157–159.

Bodnar, R. J., Kelly, D. D., Spiaggia, A., Ehrenberg, C., and Glusman, M. (1978a). Dose-dependent reductions by naloxone of analgesia induced by cold-water stress. *Pharmacol. Biochem. and Behav.,* **8**, 667–672.

Bodnar, R. J., Kelly, D. D., Spiaggia, A., and Glusman, M. (1978b). Biphasic alterations of nociceptive thresholds induced by food deprivation. *Physiol. Psychol.,* **6**, 391–395.

Bodnar, R. J., Kelly, D. D., Steiner, S. S., and Glusman, M. (1978c). Stress-produced analgesia and morphine-produced analgesia: lack of cross-tolerance. *Pharmacol. Biochem. and Behav.*, **8**, 661–666.

Bodnar, R. J., Glusman, M., Brutus, M., Spiaggia, A., and Kelly, D. D. (1979). Analgesia induced by cold-water stress: attenuation following hypophysectomy., *Physiol. and Behav.*, **23**, 53–62.

Bodnar, R. J., Abrams, G. W., Zimmerman, E. A., Krieger, D. T., Nicholson, G., and Kizer, J. S. (1980). Neonatal monosodium glutamate: effects upon analgesic responsivity and immunocytochemical ACTH/B-endorphin. *Neuroendocrinology*, **30**; 280, 284.

Cannon, J. T., Lewis, J. W., Weinberg, V. E., and Liebeskind, J. C. (1983). Evidence for the independence of brain stem mechanisms mediating analgesia induced by morphine and two forms of stress. *Brain Res.*, **269**, 231–236.

Cannon, J. T., Prieto, G. J., Lee, A., and Liebeskind, J. C. (1982). Evidence for opioid and non-opioid forms of stimulation-produced analgesia in the rat. *Brain Res.*, **243**, 315–321.

Chance, W. T. (1980). Autoanalgesia: opiate and non-opiate mechanisms. *Neurosci. and Biobehav. Rev.*, **4**, 55–67.

Chance, W. T., and Rosecrans, J. A. (1979a). Lack of cross-tolerance between morphine and autoanalgesia. *Pharmacol. Biochem. and Behav.*, **11**, 639–642.

Chance, W. T., and Rosecrans, J. A. (1979b). Lack of effect of naloxone on autoanalgesia. *Pharmacol. Biochem. and Behav.*, **11**, 643–646.

Chance, W. T., White, A. C., Krynock, G. M., and Rosecrans, J. A. (1977). Autoanalgesia: behaviorally activated antinociception. *Eur. J. Pharmacol.*, **44**, 283–284.

Chance, W. T., White, A. C., Krynock, G. M., and Rosecrans, J. A. (1978). Conditional fear-induced decreases in the binding of (^{3}H)-*N*-Leu-enkephalin to rat brain. *Brain Res.*, **141**, 371–374.

Chance, W. T., Krynock, G. M., and Rosecrans, J. A. (1979). Investigations of pituitary influences on autoanalgesia. *Psychoneuroendocrinology*, **4**, 199–205.

Chang, K. J., and Cuatrecasas, P. (1979). Multiple opiate receptors: enkephalins and morphine bind to receptors of different specificity. *J. Biol. Chem.*, **254**, 2610–2618.

Chesher, G. B., and Chan, B. (1977). Footshock induced analgesia in mice: its reversal by naloxone and cross-tolerance with morphine. *Life Sci.*, **21**, 1569–1574.

Costa, E., Guidotti, A., Hanbauer, I., Hexum, T., Saiani, L., Stine, S., and Yang, H.-Y.T (1981). 'Regulation of acetylcholine receptors by endogenous cotransmitters: studies of adrenal medulla. *Fedn Proc. Fedn Am. Socs exp. Biol.*, **40**, 160–165.

Crowley, W. R., Rodriguez-Sierra, J. F., and Komisaruk, B. R. (1977). Analgesia induced by vaginal stimulation in rats is apparently independent of a morphine-sensitive process. *Psychopharmacology*, **54**, 223–225.

D'Amour, F. E., and Smith, D. L. (1941). A method for determining loss of pain sensation. *J. Pharmacol. exp. Ther.*, **72**, 74–79.

Dennis, S. G., and Melzack, R. (1979). Comparison of phasic and tonic pain in animals, in *Advances in Pain Research and Therapy, Vol. 3* (eds J. J. Bonica, J. C. Liebeskind, and D. G. Albe-Fessard), pp. 747–760, Raven Press, New York.

Dennis, S. G., Choiniere, M., and Melzack, R. (1980). Stimulation-produced analgesia in rats: assessment by two pain tests and correlation with self-stimulation. *Exp. Neurol.*, **68**, 295–309.

Drugan, R. C., Grau, J. W., Maier, S. F., Madden, J., and Barchas, J. D. (1981). Cross-tolerance between morphine and the long term analgesic reaction to inescapable shock. *Pharmacol. Biochem. and Behav.*, **14**, 677–682.

Fields, H. L., and Basbaum, A. I. (1979). Anatomy and physiology of a descending pain control system, in *Advances in Pain Research and Therapy, Vol 3* (eds J. J. Bonica, J. C. Liebeskind, and D. G. Albe-Fessard), pp. 427–440, Raven Press, New York.

Frederickson, R. C. A., Burgis, D., and Edwards, J. D. (1977). Hyperalgesia induced by naloxone follows diurnal rhythm in responsivity to painful stimuli. *Science,* **198**, 756–759.

Giesler, G. J. Jr., and Liebeskind, J. C. (1976). Inhibition of visceral pain by electrical stimulation of the periaqueductal gray matter. *Pain,* **2**, 43–48.

Glick, S., and Crane, L. A. (1978). Opiate-like and abstinence-like effects of intracerebral histamine administration in rats. *Nature,* **273**, 547–549.

Goldstein, A., and Hilgard, E. R. (1975). Lack of influence of the morphine antagonist naloxone on hypnotic analgesia. *Proc. Natl Acad. Sci.,* **72**, 2041–2043.

Grau, J. W., Hyson, R. L., Maier, S. F., Madden, J. IV, and Barchas, J. D. (1981). Long-term stress-induced analgesia and activation of the opiate system. *Science,* **213**, 1409–1410.

Guillemin, R., Vargo, T., Rossier, J., Minick, S., Ling, N., Rivier, C., Vale, W., and Bloom, F. (1977). β-endorphin and adrenocorticotropin are secreted concomitantly by the pituitary gland. *Science,* **197**, 1367–1369.

Hayes, R. L., Bennett, G. J., Newlon, P. G., and Mayer, D. J. (1976). Analgesic effects of certain noxious and stressful manipulations in the rat. *Soc. Neurosci. Abstr.,* **2**, 939.

Hayes, R. L., Bennett, G. J., Newlon, P. G., and Mayer, D. J. (1978a). Behavioral and physiological studies of non-narcotic analgesia in the rat elicited by certain environmental stimuli. *Brain Res.,* **155**, 69–90.

Hayes, R. L., Price, D. D., Bennett, G. J., Wilcox, G. L., and Mayer, D. J. (1978b). Differential effects of spinal cord lesions on narcotic and non-narcotic suppression of nociceptive reflexes: further evidence for the physiological multiplicity of pain modulation. *Brain Res.,* **155**, 91–102.

Hökfelt, T., Ljungdahl, A., Terenius, L., Elde, R., and Nilson, G. (1977). Immunohistochemical analysis of peptide pathways possibly related to pain and analgesia: enkephalin and substance P. *Proc. Natl Acad. Sci.,* **74**, 3081–3085.

Howes, J. F., Harris, L. S., Dewey, W. L., and Voyda, C. (1969). Brain acetylcholine levels and inhibition of the tail-flick reflex in mice. *J. Pharmacol. exp. Ther.,* **169**, 23–28.

Hughes, J., Smith, T. W., Kosterlitz, H. W., Fothergill, L. A., Morgan, B. A., and Morris, H. R. (1975). Identification of two related pentapeptides from the brain with potent opiate agonist activity. *Nature,* **258**, 577–579.

Jackson, R. L., Maier, S. F., and Coon, D. J. (1979). Long-term analgesic effects of inescapable shock and learned helplessness. *Science,* **206**, 91–93.

Jacob, J. J., Tremblay, E. C., and Colombel, M-C. (1974). Facilitation de reactions nociceptives par la naloxone chez la souris et chez le rat. *Psychopharmacologia,* **37**, 217–223.

Jensen, T. S., and Smith, D. F. (1981). The role of consciousness in stress-induced analgesia. *J. Neural Trans.,* **52**, 55–60.

Kelly, D. D., Lemaire, P. A., and Leitner, D. S. (1982). Hyperalgesia and analgesia induced by the same stressor. *Soc. Neurosci. Abstr.,* **8**, 511.

Levine, J. D., Gordon, N. C., and Fields, H. L. (1978). The mechanism of placebo analgesia. *Lancet,* **ii**, 654–657.

Lewis, J. W., Cannon, J. T., and Liebeskind, J. C. (1980a). Opioid and nonopioid mechanisms of stress analgesia. *Science,* **208**, 623–625.

Lewis, J. W., Cannon, J. T., Ryan, S. M., and Liebeskind, J. C. (1980b). Behavioral pharmacology of opioid peptides, in *Role of Peptides in Neuronal Function* (ed. J. L. Barker), pp. 742–763, Marcel Dekker Inc., NY.

Lewis, J. W., Cannon, J. T., Stapleton, J. M., and Liebeskind, J. C. (1980c). Stress activates endogenous pain-inhibitory systems: opioid and nonopioid mechanisms. *Proc. West. Pharmacol. Soc.,* **23**, 85–88.

Lewis, J. W., Cannon, J. T., Liebeskind, J. C., (1983a). Involvement of central muscarinic cholinergic mechanisms in opioid stress analgesia. *Brain Res.,* **270**, 289–293.

Lewis, J. W., Cannon, J. T., Liebeskind, J. C., and Akil, H. (1981a). Alterations in brain β-endorphin immunoreactivity following acute and chronic stress. *Pain*, Suppl. 1, S263.

Lewis, J. W., Chudler, E. H., Cannon, J. T., and Liebeskind, J. C. (1981b). Hypophysectomy differentially affects morphine and stress analgesia. *Proc. West. Pharmacol. Soc.,* **24**, 323–326.

Lewis, J. W., Sherman, J. E., and Liebeskind, J. C. (1981c). Opioid and nonopioid stress analgesia: assessment of tolerance and cross-tolerance with morphine. *J. Neurosci.,* **1**, 358–363.

Lewis, J. W., Stapleton, J. M., Castiglioni, A. J. Jr., and Liebeskind, J. C. (1982a). Stimulation-produced analgesia and intrinsic mechanisms of pain suppression, in *Neuropeptides — Basic and Clinical Aspects, Proc. 11th Pfizer International Symposium* (eds G. Fink and L. J. Whalley), pp. 41–49, Churchill Livingstone, Edinburgh.

Lewis, J. W., Tordoff, M. G., Liebeskind, J. C., and Viveros, O. H. (1982b). Evidence for adrenal medullary opioid involvement in stress analgesia. *Soc. Neurosci. Abstr.,* **8**, 778.

Lewis, J. W., Tordoff, M. G., Sherman, J. E., and Liebeskind, J. C. (1982c). Adrenal medullary enkephalin-like peptides may mediate opioid stress analgesia. *Science,* **217**, 557–559.

Lewis, J. W., Terman, G. W., Watkins, L. R., Mayer, D. J., and Liebeskind, J. C. (1983b). Opioid and nonopioid mechanisms of footshock-induced analgesia: role of the spinal dorsolateral funiculus. *Brain Res.*, **267**, 139–144.

Li, C. H., and Chung, D. (1976). Isolation and structure of a triakontapeptide with opiate activity from camel pituitary glands. *Proc. Natl Acad. Sci.,* **73**, 1145–1148.

Liebeskind, J. C., Giesler, G. J. Jr., and Urca, G. (1976). Evidence pertaining to an endogenous mechanism of pain inhibition in the central nervous system, in *Sensory Functions of the Skin in Primates* (ed. Y. Zotterman), pp. 561–573, Pergamon Press, Oxford.

Livett, B. G., Dean, D. M., Whelan, L. G., Udenfriend, S., and Rossier, J. (1981). Co-release of enkephalin and catecholamines from cultured adrenal chromaffin cells. *Nature,* **289**, 317–319.

Loh, H. H., Tseng, L. F., Wei, E. and Li, C. H. (1976). β-endorphin is a potent analgesic agent. *Proc. Natl Acad. Sci. (USA),* **73**, 2895–2898.

MacLennan, A. J., Drugan, R. C., Hyson, R. L., Maier, S. F., Madden, J., and Barchas, J. D. (1982). Corticosterone: a critical factor in an opioid form of stress-induced analgesia. *Science,* **215**, 1530–1532.

Madden, J., Akil, H., Patrick, R. L., and Barchas, J. D. (1977). Stress-induced parallel changes in central opioid levels and pain responsiveness in the rat. *Nature,* **265**, 358–360.

Maier, S. F., Davies, S., Grau, J. W., Jackson, R. L., Morrison, D. H., Moye, T., Madden, J., and Barchas, J. D. (1980). Opiate antagonists and the long-term analgesic reactions induced by inescapable shock in rats. *J. Comp. Physiol. Psychol.,* **94**, 1172–1183.

Maier, S. F., Sherman, J. E., Lewis, J. W., Terman, G. W., and Liebeskind, J. C. (1983). The opioid-nonopioid nature of stress-induced analgesia and learned helplessness. *J. Exp. Psych.: Animal Behav. Processes,* **9**, 80–90.

Mayer, D. J., and Hayes, R. L. (1975). Stimulation-produced analgesia: development of tolerance and cross-tolerance to morphine. *Science,* **188**, 941–943.

Mayer, D. J., and Price, D. D. (1976). Central nervous system mechanisms of analgesia. *Pain,* **2**, 379–404.

Mayer, D. J., Wolfle, T. L., Akil, H., Carder, B., and Liebeskind, J. C. (1971). Analgesia from electrical stimulation in the brainstem of the rat. *Science,* **174**, 1351–1354.

Mayer, D. J., Price, D. D., Rafii, A., and Barber, J. (1976). Acupuncture hypoalgesia: evidence for activation of a central control system as a mechanism of action', in *Advances in Pain Research and Therapy, Vol. 1* (eds J. J. Bonica and D. Albe-Fessard), pp. 751–754, Raven Press, NY.

McGivern, R. F., Berka, C., Berntson, G. G., Walker, J. M., and Sandman, C. A. (1979). Effect of naloxone on analgesia induced by food deprivation. *Life Sci.,* **25**, 885–888.

McGivern, R. F., and Berntson, G. G. (1980). Mediation of diurnal fluctuations in pain sensitivity in the rat by food intake patterns: reversal by naloxone. *Science,* **210**, 210–211.

Miczek, K. A., Thompson, M. L., and Shuster, L. (1982). Opioid-like analgesia in defeated mice. *Science,* **215**, 1520–1522.

Millan, M. J., Przewlocki, R., and Herz, A. (1980). A non-β-endorphinergic adenohypophyseal mechanism is essential for an analgetic response to stress. *Pain,* **8**, 343–353.

Millan, M. J., Tsang, Y. F., Przewlocki, R., Hollt, V., and Herz, A. (1981). The influence of foot-shock stress upon brain, pituitary, and spinal cord pools of immunoreactive dynorphin in rats. *Neurosci. Lett.,* **24**, 75–79.

Nelson, L. R., Lewis, J. W., Liebeskind, J. C., Branch, B. J., and Taylor, A. N. (1982). Fetal exposure to ethanol potentiates opioid stress analgesia in adult rats. *Soc. Neurosci. Abstr.,* **8**, 596.

Oleson, T. D., Twombly, D. A., and Liebeskind, J. C. (1978). Effects of pain-attenuating brain stimulation and morphine on electrical activity in the raphe nuclei of the awake rat. *Pain,* **4**, 211–230.

Oliveras, J. L., Besson, J. M., Guilbaud, G., and Liebeskind, J. C. (1974). Behavioral and electrophysiological evidence of pain inhibition from midbrain stimulation in the cat. *Exp. Brain Res.,* **20**, 32–44.

Oliveras, J. L., Hosobuchi, Y., Redjemi, F., Guilbaud, G., and Besson, J. M. (1977). Opiate antagonist, naloxone, strongly reduces analgesia induced by stimulation of a raphe nucleus (centralis inferior). *Brain Res.,* **120**, 221–229.

Pedigo, N. W., and Dewey, W. L. (1981). Acetylcholine induced antinociception; comparisons to opiate analgesia, in *Cholinergic Mechanisms: Phylogenetic Aspects, Central and Peripheral Synapses, and Clinical Significance, Adv. in Behav. Biol. Vol. 25* (eds G. Pepeu and H. Ladinsky), pp. 795–807, Plenum Press, New York.

Penner, E. R., Terman, G. W., and Liebeskind, J. C. (1982). Cross-tolerance between opioid mediated stimulation-produced and stress-induced analgesia. *Soc. Neurosci. Abstr.,* **8**, 619.

Pert, A. and Maxey, G. (1975). Asymmetrical cross-tolerance between morphine and scopolamine induced antinociception in the primate: differential sites of action. *Psychopharmacologia,* **44**, 139–145.

Pert, A., and Walter, M. (1976). Comparison between naloxone reversal of morphine and electrical stimulation induced analgesia in the rat mesencephalon. *Life Sci.,* **19**, 1023–1032.

Pomeranz, B., and Chiu, D. (1976). Naloxone blockade of acupuncture analgesia: endorphins implicated. *Life Sci.*, **19**, 1757–1762.

Prieto, G. J., Cannon, J. T., and Liebeskind, J. C. (1983). N. raphe magnus lesions disrupt stimulation-produced analgesia from ventral but not dorsal midbrain areas in the rat. *Brain Res.*, **261**, 53–57.

Reynolds, D. V. (1969). Surgery in the rat during electrical analgesia induced by focal brain stimulation. *Science,* **164**, 444–445.

Rossier, J., French, E. D., Rivier, C., Ling, N., Guillemin, R., and Bloom, F. E. (1977a). Foot-shock induced stress increases β-endorphin levels in blood but not brain. *Nature,* **270**, 618–620.

Rossier, J., Vargo, T. M., Minick, S., Ling, N., Bloom, F. E., and Guillemin, R. (1977b). Regional dissociation of β-endorphin and enkephalin contents in rat brain and pituitary. *Proc. Natl. Acad. Sci.,* **74**, 5162–5165.

Rossier, J., Guillemin, R., and Bloom, F. E. (1978). Foot-shock induced stress decreases leu^5-enkephalin immunoreactivity in rat hypothalamus. *Eur. J. Pharmacol.,* **48**, 465–466.

Saria, A., Wilson, S. P., Molnar, A., Viveros, O. H., and Lembeck, F. (1980). Substance P and opiate-like peptides in human adrenal medulla. *Neurosci. Lett.,* **20**, 195–200.

Satoh, M., Akaike, A., Nakazawa, T., and Takagi, H. (1980). Evidence for involvement of separate mechanisms in the production of analgesia by electrical stimulation of the nucleus reticularis paragigantocellularis and nucleus raphe magnus in the rat. *Brain Res.,* **194**, 525–529.

Schultzberg, M., Lundberg, J. M., Hökfelt, T., Terenius, L., Brandt, J., Elde, R. P., and Goldstein, M. (1978). Enkephalin-like immunoreactivity in gland cells and nerve terminals of the adrenal medulla. *Neurosci.,* **3**, 1169–1186.

Schwartz, J. C., Barbin, G., Duchemin, A. M., Garbarg, M., Pollard, H., and Quach, T. T. (1981). Functional role of histamine in the brain, in *Neuropharmacology of Central Nervous System and Behavioral Disorders* (ed. G. C. Palmer), pp. 539–570, Academic Press, NY.

Selye, H. (1956). *The Stress of Life*, McGraw-Hill Book Co. Inc., New York.

Sherman, J. E., and Liebeskind, J. C. (1980). An endorphinergic, centrifugal substrate of pain modulation: recent findings, current concepts, and complexities, in *Pain* (ed. J. J. Bonica), pp. 191–204, Raven Press, NY.

Taylor, A. N., Branch, B. J., Liu, S. H., and Kokka, N. (1982). Long-term effects of fetal ethanol exposure on pituitary-adrenal response to stress. *Pharmac. Biochem. and Behav.,* **16**, 585–589.

Terman, G. W., Lewis, J. W., and Liebeskind, J. C. (1981). Monoaminergic mechanisms of stress analgesia. *Soc. Neurosci. Abstr.,* **7**, 879.

Terman, G. W., Lewis, J. W., and Liebeskind, J. C. (1982a). Role of the biogenic amines in stress analgesia. *Proc. West. Pharmacol. Soc.,* **25**, 7–10.

Terman, G. W., Lewis, J. W., and Liebeskind, J. C. (1982b). Evidence for the involvement of histamine in stress analgesia. *Soc. Neurosci. Abstr.,* **8**, 619.

Terman, G. W., Lewis, J. W., and Liebeskind, J. C. (1983a). Opioid and nonopioid mechanisms of stress analgesia: lack of cross-tolerance between stressors. *Brain Res.,* **260**, 147–150.

Terman, G. W., Lewis, J. W., and Liebeskind, J. C. (1983b). The sensitivity of opioid mediated stress analgesia to narcotic antagonists. *Proc. West. Pharmacol. Soc.*, **26**, 53–56.

Torda, C. (1978). Effects of recurrent postnatal pain-related stressful events on opiate receptor-endogenous ligand system. *Psychoneuroendocrinology,* **3**, 85–91.

Urca, G., and Liebeskind, J. C. (1979). Electrophysiological indices of opiate action in awake and anaesthetized rats. *Brain Res.,* **161**, 162–166.

Viveros, O. H., Diliberto, E. J. Jr., Hazum, E., and Chang, K.-J. (1979). Opiate-like materials in the adrenal medulla: evidence for storage and secretion with catecholamines. *Molec. Pharmac.*, **16**, 1101–1108.

Viveros, O. H., Diliberto, E. J. Jr., Hazum, E., and Chang, K.-J. (1980). Enkephalins as possible adrenomedullary hormones: storage, secretion, and regulation of synthesis, in *Neural Peptides and Neuronal Comunication* (eds E. Costa and M. Trabucchi), pp. 191–204, Raven Press, NY.

Viveros, O. H., and Wilson, S. P. (1983). The adrenal chromaffin cell as a model to study the co-secretion of enkephalins and catecholamines. *J. Autonom. Nerv. Syst.*, **7**, 41–58.

Wamsley, J. K., Lewis, M. S., Young, S. III, and Kuhar, M. J. (1981). Autoradiographic localization of muscarinic cholinergic receptors in rat brainstem. *J. Neurosci.*, **1**, 176–191.

Watkins, L. R., Griffin, G., Leichnitz, G. R., and Mayer, D. J. (1980). The somatotopic organization of the nucleus raphe magnus and surrounding brain stem structures as revealed by HRP slow-release gels. *Brain Res.*, **181**, 1–15.

Watkins, L. R., and Mayer, D. J. (1982). The organization of endogenous opiate and nonopiate pain control systems. *Science,* **216**, 1185–1192.

Watkins, L. R., Young, E., Kinsheck, I., and Mayer, D. J. (1981). Effects of n raphe alatus (NRA) lesions and periaqueductal gray (PAG) lesions on footshock induced analgesia (FSIA) and classically conditioned analgesia. *Soc. Neurosci. Abstr.*, **7**, 340.

Watkins, L. R., Cobelli, D. A., Faris, P., Aceto, M. D., and Mayer, D. J. (1982a). Opiate vs. non-opiate footshock induced analgesia (FSIA): the body region shocked is a critical factor. *Brain Res.*, **242**, 299–308.

Watkins, L. R., Cobelli, D. A., and Mayer, D. J. (1982b). Opiate vs. non-opiate footshock analgesia (FSIA): descending and intraspinal components. *Brain Res.*, **245**, 97–106.

Watkins, L. R., Cobelli, D. A., Newsome, H. H., and Mayer, D. J. (1982c). Footshock induced analgesia is dependent neither on pituitary nor sympathetic activation. *Brain Res.*, **245**, 81–96.

Watson, S. J., Akil, H., and Barchas, J. D. (1979). Immunohistochemical and biochemical studies of the enkephalins, β-endorphin and related peptides, in *Endorphins in Mental Health Research* (eds E. Usdin, W. E. Bunney Jr., and N. S. Kline), Oxford University Press, NY.

Wilson, S. P., Chang, K.-J., and Viveros, O. H. (1980). Synthesis of enkephalins by adrenal medullary chromaffin cells: reserpine increased incorporation of radiolabelled amino acids. *Proc. Natl Acad. Sci. USA.*, **77**, 4364–4368.

Yaksh, T. L., and Rudy, T. A. (1978). Narcotic analgetics: CNS sites and mechanisms of action as revealed by intracerebral injection techniques. *Pain,* **4**, 299–359.

Yaksh, T. L., Yeung, J. C., and Rudy, T. A. (1976). An inability to antagonize with naloxone the elevated thresholds resulting from electrical stimulation of the mesencephalic central gray. *Life Sci.*, **18**, 1193–1198.

Zorman, G., Hentall, I. D., Adams, J. E., and Fields, H. L. (1981). Naloxone-reversible analgesia produced by microstimulation in the rat medulla. *Brain Res.*, **219**, 137–148.

Stress-induced Analgesia
Edited by M. D. Tricklebank and G. Curzon

CHAPTER 6

Anti-nociception induced by brief footshock: characteristics and roles of 5-hydroxytryptamine and dopamine

P. H. Hutson, G. Curzon and M. D. Tricklebank

INTRODUCTION

It is now well established that a wide variety of stressful or painful stimuli including inescapable footshock (Madden *et al.*, 1977), centrifugal rotation (Hayes *et al.*, 1978), cold water swims (Bodnar *et al.*, 1979), immobilization (Bhattacharya *et al.*, 1978), injection of hypertonic saline (Hayes *et al.*, 1978), or 2-deoxyglucose (Bodnar *et al.*, 1979) induce short lasting (typically 30 min) reductions in responsiveness to subsequent noxious stimuli. These reductions are often quite substantial and have been compared to the effects of 10 mg/kg morphine (Bodnar *et al.*, 1978a). The phenomenon has been termed stress-induced analgesia or anti-nociception. However, it cannot be induced by all stressful stimuli. Thus Hayes *et al.* (1978) showed that while most noxious and some non-noxious stimuli provoked anti-nociception, other stimuli, i.e. exposure to ether vapour or horizontal oscillation did not.

The underlying mechanisms involved in this behavioural response to stress need to be clarified. However, the mechanisms involved in stress-induced anti-nociception appear complex and factors such as shock duration, region of the body shocked, and exposure to noxious stimuli before shock are important variables. This chapter describes some investigations on the role of endogenous opioids, 5-hydroxytryptamine, and dopamine in relation to some of these factors.

METHODS

While this chapter does not have the structure of a formal research paper, a methodological section is included because it is becoming increasingly apparent that details of experimental design can have profound effects on stress-induced anti-nociceptive phenomena.

In all experiments, male Sprague-Dawley rats (Charles-River UK, Ltd), weight range 205 ± 12 g were used. They were singly housed on a 12 h light–dark cycle (white light on 06.00 h) and allowed food and water *ad lib* for approximately seven days. Responsiveness to noxious thermal stimuli was assessed using either the paw-lick method essentially as described by Hayes *et al.* (1978) or the tail-flick test (similar to that described by D'Amour and Smith, 1941). The following modifications to these methods were used.

Procedure 1. Latency to lick the paws or flick the tail was determined before (L1) and after (L2) exposing rats to a period of footshock. Control animals were returned to their home cages between latency measurements. Percentage anti-nociception score was calculated from (L2/L1) × 100.
Procedure 2. Rats were used as their own controls. Thus paw-lick or tail-flick latencies were determined initially (L1), 30 s after replacement in the home cage (L2) and after exposure to footshock (L3). Percentage anti-nociception score was determined from the ratio (L3/L2) × 100 for shocked rats and (L2/L1) × 100 to give a non-shock control score. In some experiments, additional latency mesurements were made at various times after shock. These values were divided by the L2 value to obtain percentage anti-nociception scores for that time point.
Procedure 3. When rats were shocked for 30 min, each latency (i.e. L1, L2, and L3) was determined in triplicate at 10 s intervals and the means used to calculate percentage anti-nociception score as above.

Footshock was applied as follows: the rats were placed in an aluminium box (240 × 210 × 90 mm high) with a front wall of clear perspex. The roof was low enough to prevent the animals from minimizing shock by rearing. The floor was a grid of 4 mm diameter stainless steel bars spaced 14 mm between centres, through which shock was delivered via a constant current shock source (shock pulses of 5 s with less than 1 s intervals between pulses).

CHARACTERISTICS OF THE ANTI-NOCICEPTIVE RESPONSE TO BRIEF FOOTSHOCK

Using the paw-lick method it was found that 30 s of 1 mA footshock caused marked anti-nociception when this was measured immediately after the termination of shock. This effect was approximately doubled when the current was increased to 2 mA (Figure 6.1). These responses decayed on repeated testing and initially decayed more rapidly after 2 mA than after 1 mA shock so that the scores of rats shocked at 1 or 2 mA s were comparable with each other 5 and 10 min after termination of shock (Figure 6.1). Results in Figure 6.2 show

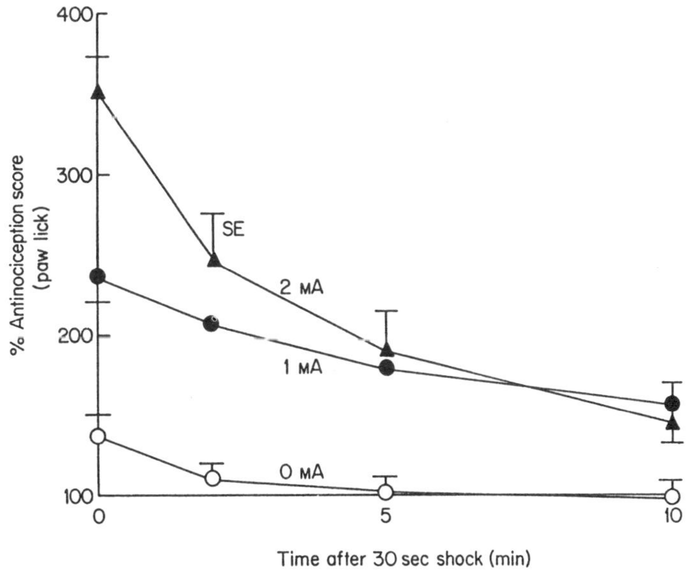

FIGURE 6.1 Time course of anti-nociceptive response to brief (30 s) footshock (1 or 2 mA). Values are means +s.e.m, 6–7 rats per group. Percentage analgesia (anti-nociception) scores were obtained using Procedure 2. All post-shock percentage analgesia scores, with the exception of the 10 min value for rats shocked at 2 mA were significantly different from pre-shock control values, $p < 0.05$ (Student's *t* test). All post-shock values whether at 1 or 2 mA were significantly different from those of non-shocked rats at the same times, $p < 0.05$ (Student's *t* test).

that when a constant intensity of footshock was applied, varying the shock duration between 10 and 120 s did not significantly alter the magnitude of the nociceptive effect when measured immediately after termination of shock.

Riffee *et al.* (1979) have reported that the variability of behavioural responses to drugs could be reduced by repeated daily handling. However, such an effect was not convincingly apparent using rats which were handled and injected with 0.9% NaCl daily for 3 days before anti-nociceptive testing (Table 6.1).

Pain sensitivity in the absence of stress has been shown to vary with the time of day being greater in the dark period (Frederickson *et al.*, 1977) and is associated with lower concentrations of forebrain 5-hydroxytryptamine (Schlosberg and Harvey, 1978) and whole brain total opioid activity (Wesche and Frederickson, 1979). Also, Puglisi-Allegra *et al.* (1982) found circadian variations of shock-induced anti-nociception in mice with larger effects on tail-flick latencies during the light phase. We find that rats kept on a 12 h light–dark cycle show less anti-nociception in response to brief footshock

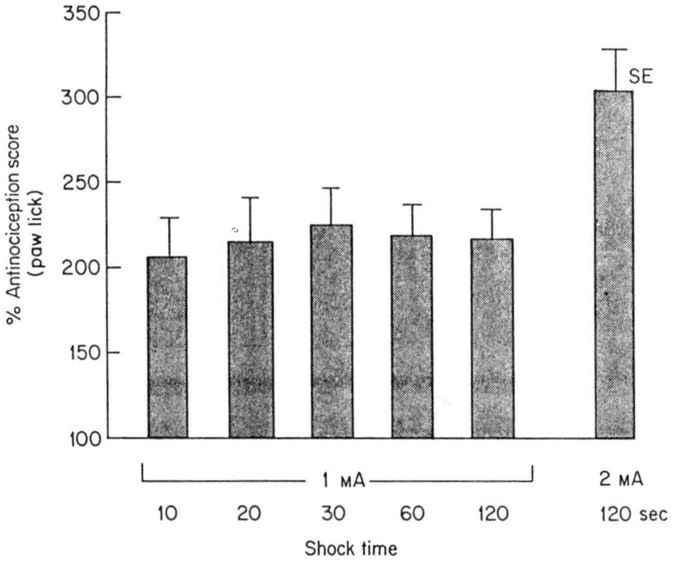

FIGURE 6.2 Effect of shock duration on percentage anti-nociception score. Values are means +s.e.m, 6–7 rats per group. Scores were determined using Procedure 2.

TABLE 6.1 Effect of previous handling on the increase of percentage anti-nociception score following brief footshock (1 mA, 30 s).

Treatment	Percentage anti-nociception score (paw-lick method)	
	Non-shock	Shock
Non-handled	93.9 ± 22.4 (10)	182.5 ± 40.5 (10)*
Handled	100.9 ± 20.7 (9)	190.8 ± 26.3 (8)*

Values are means ± s.d. Number of rats in brackets. Percentage anti-nociception score was calculated from paw-lick latency using Procedure 2.

*$p < 0.001$ compared with non-shock control values (Student's *t* test).

during the late red and early white phases than during the late white and early red phases (Figure 6.3).

Repeated exposure to stress has been shown to produce various effects on stress-induced anti-nociception. Thus, if mild footshock is paired with an unconditioned stimulus, e.g. the shock chamber (Chance *et al.*, 1977; Hayes *et al.*, 1978) or an audible tone (Oliverio and Castellano, 1982) than anti-nociception occurs if the animals are re-exposed to the unconditioned stimulus 24h later. However, it has also been reported that daily exposure to stress decreases the subsequent nociceptive response (Madden *et al.*, 1977;

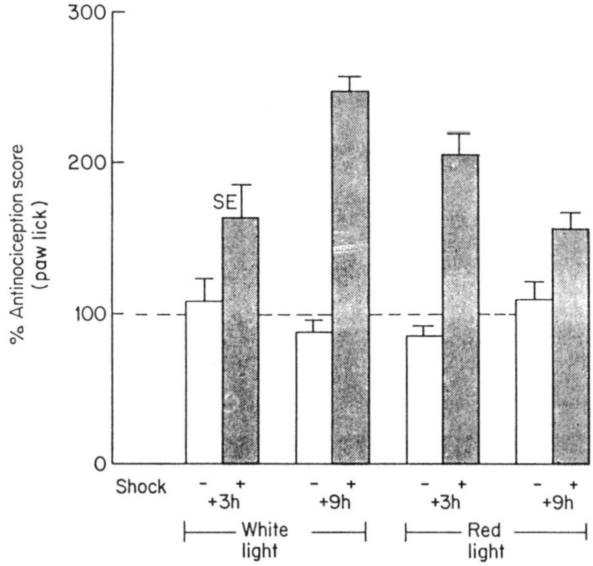

FIGURE 6.3 Circadian variation of percentage anti-nociception score in response to brief footshock (1 mA, 30 s). Values are means +s.e.m., 9–11 rats per group. Separate groups of rats were used for non-shock and shock treatments. Scores were calculated according to Procedure 1. Open columns, non-shocked rats, closed closed columns, shocked rats. There was no significant difference of percentage analgesia score in non-shocked rats at different periods of the light : dark cycle. Percentage analgesia scores of shocked rats were significantly greater ($p < 0.02$) than values for non-shock controls. Percentage analgesia scores were significantly lower ($p < 0.001$) in the early white and late red phases than in the late white and early red phases.

Bodnar *et al.*, 1978b) and more recently Lai and Chan (1981) have shown that even in the absence of stress, repeated weekly exposure of rats to a hot-plate gradually decreases paw-lick latency.

Figure 6.4(a) shows the results of our own investigations. In this experiment, rats were subjected to Procedure 1, once a day for five days, i.e. both pre- and post-shock analgesia values were obtained each day and used to calculate per cent analgesia score. The latter value was significantly greater than that of non-shocked rats only on the first day. By the fifth day, values for shocked and non-shocked rats were virtually identical. Although this is superficially reminiscent of the development of tolerance, Figure 6.4(b) shows that post-shock latencies (L2) expressed as percentages of corresponding L2 values for control rats which had been put through the same procedure each

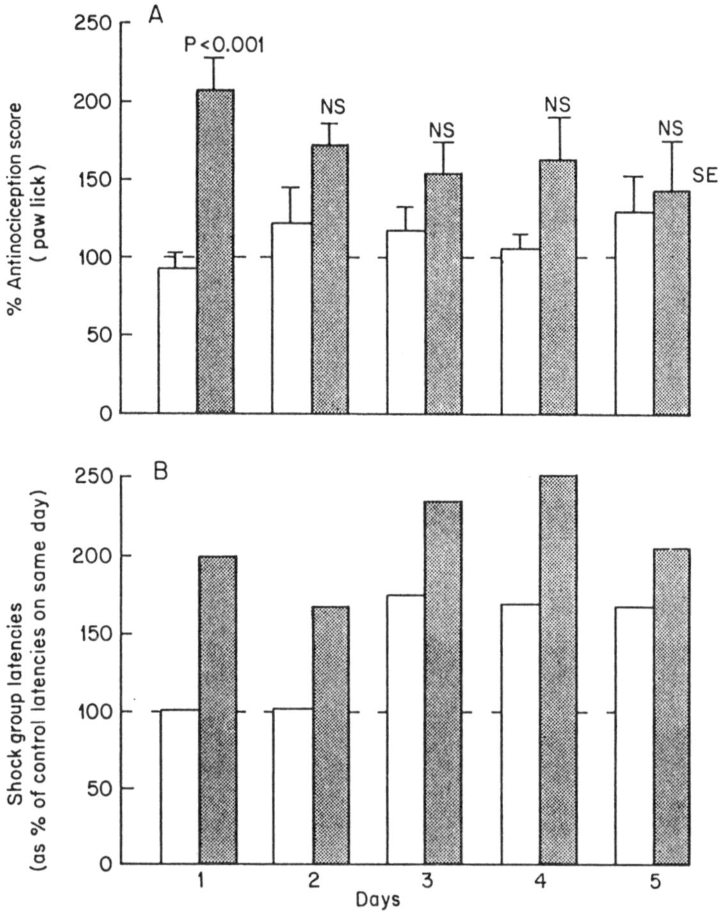

FIGURE 6.4 Effect of footshock (1 mA, 30s) repeated daily on (A) percentage anti-nociception score: Values are means +s.e.m., 6–8 rats per group. Scores were determined by Procedure 1. Open columns, non-shock controls; closed columns, shocked rats. (B) paw-lick latencies: Open columns show the latency values (L1) obtained before shock on the day indicated of rats shocked on previous days. They are divided by L1 values of the control animals. Closed columns show the latency values (L2) obtained after shock on the day indicated of rats shocked on previous days. They are divided by L2 values of the control animals.

day (except for shock-exposure) remained high throughout the five-day period. Figure 6.4(b) also shows that pre-shock latencies (L1) of the rats which had been shocked on previous days were greater than the corresponding L1 values for the controls from the third day onwards. Thus, percent analgesia scores of the shocked animals *appeared* to decline over the five-day period of the experiment largely because they were obtained by dividing the L2 values by the above increased L1 values. These results suggest that after two daily shock exposures the anti-nociceptive effect of the shock is largely maintained 24 h later. A possible explanation of this result is that an association is established between the pre-shock paw-lick test and subsequent shock.

The above result may be contrasted with the rapid attenuation of the anti-nociceptive effect of shock when a series of paw-lick tests is applied after a single brief shock period (Figure 6.1). It may be that in the latter circumstances, the train of tests of nociception not interspersed with periods of shock exposure serves to attenuate the association between test and shock.

An interpretation of this kind implies that learning processes may be involved in the analgesic effect of brief shock and that this depends on exposure to the test of nociception before shock. Results in Table 6.2 clearly indicate such a dependence as 30 s shock no longer caused increased latency when the pre-shock tail-flick test was omitted. However, there was no such dependence on pre-shock testing when rats were shocked for 30 min, perhaps because the association between noxious heat and shock was disrupted by the prolonged period of footshock (Tricklebank *et al.*, 1984a).

Table 6.2 Effect of pre-shock anti-nociceptive testing on post-shock tail-flick latency.

	Shock time (min)	Tail flick latency (s) Pre-shock	Post-shock
Pre-shock test (11)	0.5	4.57 ± 1.00	8.89 ± 2.01**
No pre-shock test (11)	0.5		4.56 ± 1.36†
Pre-shock test (7)	30	3.27 ± 0.59	5.70 ± 1.84*
No pre-shock test (8)	30		6.63 ± 1.87

Values are means ± s.d. Number of rats in brackets. Tail-flick latency was determined immediately before (L1) and/or after (L2) footshock (2 mA, 30 s). When rats were shocked for 30 min, tail-flick latencies for L1 and L2 were then done in triplicate at 10 s intervals and the mean values used. $^*p < 0.01$, $^{**}p < 0.001$ compared with L1 values using Student's *t* test for paired observations. $^\dagger p < 0.001$ compared with L2 of pre-shock test group (Student's *t* test) (data from Tricklebank *et al.*, 1984a).

ENDOGENOUS OPIOIDS

Many previous studies on the role of endogenous opioids in stress-induced anti-nociception led to conflicting results. Madden *et al.* (1977) found that inescapable footshock increased both tail-flick latency and brain opioid peptide concentration and that repeated daily exposure to the shock led to attenuation of both effects. Chance *et al.* (1977) found decreased brain opioid binding and increased anti-nociception when rats were exposed to classical conditioning procedures. Chronic treatment with naltrexone was found to increase footshock-induced anti-nociception (Amir and Amit, 1979). Acute treatment with naltrexone (Maier *et al.*, 1980) or naloxone prevented the anti-nociceptive response to stress (Chesher and Chan, 1977; Bodnar *et al.*, 1978a; Buckett, 1979; Shimizu *et al.*, 1981) although in the study by Bodnar *et al.* only a 50% reduction of anti-nociception was obtained with an extremely large dose of naloxone and Buckett (1979) found no cross-tolerance between naloxone reversible stress-induced anti-nociception and that due to morphine which suggested that two opioid mechanisms were present. In contrast, a lack of involvement of the endogenous opioids was suggested by the failure of a wide range of doses of naloxone to affect anti-nociception induced by various stressors (Hayes *et al.*, 1978; Bodnar *et al.*, 1979; Chance and Rosecrans, 1979a; Rodgers and Deacon, 1981). Furthermore, while tolerance to the anti-nociceptive effects of both stress and morphine were demonstrated, there was no cross-tolerance between these treatments (Bodnar *et al.*, 1978b; Chance and Rosecrans, 1979b) which suggested the involvement of a non-opiate mechanism in the effect of stress. Table 6.3 shows that in agreement with these studies, naloxone at doses between 1 and 20 mg/kg did not attenuate anti-nociception induced by brief footshock.

Table 6.3 Effect of naloxone on anti-nociception induced by brief footshock (1 mA, 30 s).

Treatment	Percentage anti-nociception score (paw-lick method)	
	Non-shock	Shock
Saline	102.3 ± 36.4	219.6 ± 67.7
Naloxone (mg/kg)		
1	77.7 ± 20.9	244.9 ± 81.4
5	102.8 ± 28.6	228.1 ± 33.9
10	93.1 ± 29.6	246.7 ± 62.5
20	98.1 ± 17.5	284.5 ± 78.3

Values are means ± s.d. 6 rats/group. Naloxone was given i.p. 30 min before shock. Percentage anti-nociception scores were determined by Procedure 2. (Data from Tricklebank *et al.*, 1982.)

Controversy about the involvement of the endogenous opioids in stress-induced anti-nociception was clarified by Lewis *et al.* (1980) who showed that both opioid and non-opioid mechanisms were involved dependent on the temporal characteristics of the stress. Thus, anti-nociception due to 3 min footshock was unaffected by naloxone, whereas that induced by more prolonged footshock (i.e. 30 min shock) was prevented. Similar results were also found with naltrexone by Grau *et al.* (1981). Further evidence for the existence of both opioid and non-opioid mechanisms was provided by Lewis *et al.* (1981) who showed that tolerance developed to the naloxone-sensitive, but not the naloxone insensitive anti-nociception and that morphine tolerant-rats could show cross-tolerance only to the naloxone-sensitive anti-nociception. In agreement with Lewis *et al.* (1980) and Grau *et al.* (1981) we also found (Tricklebank *et al.*, 1984a) that anti-nociception following prolonged (30 min), but not brief (30 s) footshock was attenuated by a low dose of naloxone (Table 6.4).

TABLE 6.4 Effect of naloxone (1 mg/kg) on anti-nociception induced by brief or prolonged footshock (2 mA).

		Percentage anti-nociception score (tail-flick method)	
Shock time (min)	Treatment	Non-shock	Shock
0.5	Vehicle	106.8 ± 17.9	243.1 ± 32.8**
0.5	Naloxone	99.2 ± 21.9	249.1 ± 65.6**
30	Vehicle	108.9 ± 23.8	149.8 ± 19.3*
30	Naloxone	105.9 ± 11.9	115.8 ± 19.3†

Values are means ± s.d. Number of rats, 7–9 group. Naloxone or vehicle was given i.p. 30 min before shock (2 mA). *$p < 0.01$, **$p < 0.001$ compared with non-shocked rats. †$p < 0.01$ compared with vehicle-treated shocked rats using Student's *t*test. Percentage anti-nociception score was determined by Procedure 2 for rats shocked for 30 s and by Procedure 3 for rats shocked for 30 min. (Data from Tricklebank *et al.*, 1984a)

However, it would appear that the opioid involvement in footshock-induced anti-nociception is more complicated than indicated by these observations as Watkins *et al.* (1982) showed that brief footshock applied to the forepaws produced naloxone reversible anti-nociception but when it was applied to the hindpaws or to all four paws the anti-nociception was not sensitive to naloxone and did not show cross-tolerance with morphine.

5-HYDROXYTRYPTAMINE

Non-opioid mechanisms of stress-induced anti-nociception have hitherto been less extensively studied, though evidence for roles of central monoamine pathways in pain sensitivity and in the anti-nociceptive activity of morphine is abundant (Tenen, 1967; Messing *et al.*, 1976; Yaksh and Wilson, 1979; Ogren and Holm, 1980).

Bhattacharya *et al.* (1978) reported that anti-nociception induced by 4 h immobilization was significantly attenuated by depleting brain 5-hydroxytryptamine with the tryptophan hydroxylase inhibitor *p*-chlorophenylalanine or by the 5-hydroxytryptamine neurotoxin 5,7-dihydroxytryptamine. In support of this work, yohimbine (Chance and Schechter, 1979), cyproheptadine

(Kulkarni, 1980), or methysergide (Shimizu *et al.*, 1981) (which among other actions are thought to block 5-hydroxytryptamine receptors) attenuated the anti-nociceptive response to a variety of prolonged stressful stimuli.

However, in contrast to these results we found that *p*-chlorophenylalanine treatment enhanced the anti-nociceptive effect of brief footshock as determined by the tail-flick or paw-lick methods (Table 6.5) (Tricklebank *et al.*, 1982). Similarly, the effect of shock on the anti-nociceptive score was enhanced when spinal cord 5-hydroxytryptamine was specifically depleted by injection of 5,7-dihydroxytryptamine either into the cord itself or into the raphé magnus (Table 6.6). Depletion of forebrain, but not spinal cord 5-hydroxytryptamine, by injecting 5,7-dihydroxytryptamine into the medial raphé was without effect (Table 6.7; Hutson *et al.*, 1982).

The above results indicate an involvement of descending 5-hydroxytryptamine pathways in the anti-nociceptive response to brief footshock but suggest an inverse relationship between 5-hydroxytryptamine and anti-nociception which contrasts with the generally accepted positive relationship between brain 5-hydroxytryptamine and pain threshold in the absence of prior stressful experiences (see references at the beginning of this section). They also contrast with previous studies on anti-nociception induced by more prolonged stress (Bhattacharya *et al.*, 1978; Chance and Schechter, 1979; Kulkarni, 1979; Shimizu *et al.*, 1981). Since Lewis *et al.* (1980) previously showed that the duration of stress has a critical effect on the nature of the resultant anti-nociception we therefore compared the effects of 5-hydroxytryptamine depletion on anti-nociception induced by brief and prolonged footshock.

Table 6.8 shows that the involvement of 5-hydroxytryptamine in shock-induced anti-nociception (like that of opioids) depends on shock duration. Thus *p*-chlorophenylalanine enhanced anti-nociception due to 30 s footshock but decreased anti-nociception due to 30 min footshock. These results imply that some intermediate duration of shock might have an anti-nociceptive effect which was unaffected by the drug. Indeed Terman *et al.* (1982) found that *p*-chlorophenylalanine had no effect on anti-nociception induced by 3 min footshock. However, with the experimental design they used only a decreased effect of shock on anti-nociception would have been detectable. This comment also applies to the work of Jensen and Smith (1982a) who reported that *p*-chlorophenylalanine did not affect anti-nociception induced by 20 s footshock.

Further evidence that anti-nociception induced by brief footshock is inversely related to 5-hydroxytryptamine availability was provided by experiments with drugs that increase its extraneuronal concentration. Thus, 30 min after giving either *p*-chloroamphetamine or fenfluramine to enhance 5-hydroxytryptamine release (Trulson and Jacobs, 1976) the anti-nociceptive effect of brief footshock was markedly reduced (Table 6.9). Similar results were

TABLE 6.5 Effect of *p*-chlorophenylalanine on brain 5-hydroxytryptamine concentration and anti-nociception induced by brief shock (1 mA, 30 s).

Anti-nociception test	Treatment	Percentage anti-nociception score		Brain 5-hydroxytryptamine concentration (ng/g)
		Non-shock	Shock	
Paw-lick	Saline	101.8 ± 44.2	211.8 ± 54.9**	690 ± 50
	p-chlorophenylalanine	97.3 ± 23.8	292.8 ± 95.4**,†	130 ± 20††
Tail-flick	Saline	112.8 ± 22.6	156.0 ± 22.6*	nd
	p-chlorophenylalanine	123.1 ± 22.1	214.9 ± 33.7**,††	nd

nd = not determined

Values are means ± s.d. Number of rats, 9–10/group. *p*-Chlorophenylalanine methyl ester HCl 150 mg/kg i.p. or saline was given daily for 3 days and rats tested 24 h after the last injection. 5-Hydroxytryptamine was determined after serial tail-flick and paw-lick determination by the method of Curzon and Green (1970). *$p < 0.01$, **$p < 0.001$ compared with non-shocked rats. †$p < 0.05$, ††$p < 0.001$ compared with saline-treated shocked rats using Student's *t* test. Percentage anti-nociception scores were calculated by Procedure 1. (Data from Tricklebank *et al.*, 1982.)

TABLE 6.6 Effects of intraspinal and raphé magnus 5,7-dihydroxytryptamine injection on regional 5-hydroxytryptamine concentration and anti-nociception induced by brief shock (1 mA, 30 s).

Treatment	Percentage anti-nociception score (paw-lick method)		5-hydroxytryptamine concentration (ng/g)		
	Non-shock	Shock	Lumbar cord	Thoracic cord	Pons + medulla oblongata
Spinal injection					
Vehicle	92.5 ± 37.8 (5)	187.4 ± 57.5 (5)†	538 ± 74 (5)	211 ± 43 (5)	220 ± 11 (5)
5,7-dihydroxytryptamine	102.4 ± 19.2 (11)	261.7 ± 59.1 (9)*,††	95 ± 51** (9)	112 ± 51** (9);	259 ± 62 (8)
% Change			−82%	−47%	+17%
Raphé magnus injection					
Vehicle	98.4 ± 17.4 (9)	188.5 ± 20.1 (9) ††	450 ± 63 (9)	314 ± 45 (9)	338 ± 27 (9)
5,7-dihydroxytryptamine	91.3 ± 22.3 (6)	298 ± 65.9 (6)**††	164 ± 81** (6)	165 ± 59** (6)	298 ± 54 (6)
% Change			−63%	−47%	−12%

Values are means ± s.d. Number of rats in brackets. Rats were pretreated with desmethylimipramine (25 mg/kg i.p.). 60 min later, after anaesthesia with sagatal BDH (45 mg/kg i.p.) they were injected between L6 and S1 vertebrae with 25 μg 5,7-dihydroxytryptamine free base in 25 μl vehicle (0.9% NaCl containing 1 mg/ml ascorbic acid). Raphé magnus lesions were produced by injecting 8 μg 5,7-dihydroxytryptamine free base in 1 μl vehicle using coordinates from Pellegrino *et al.* (1979) (rostral-caudal −8.2 mm, posterior to bregma; medio-lateral, 0.0 mm; dorsal-ventral, 7.5 mm below the surface of the dura) at 1 μl/min. Percentage anti-nociception scores were determined 9 days later by paw-lick (Procedure 2). 5-hydroxytryptamine was determined by HPLC (Curzon *et al.*, 1981). †$p < 0.02$, ††$p < 0.001$ compared with non-shock controls; *$p < 0.05$, **$p < 0.001$ compared with vehicle-treated rats. (Data from Hutson *et al.*, 1982.)

Table 6.7 Effect of medial raphé 5,7-dihydroxytryptamine injection on regional 5-hydroxytryptamine concentration and anti-nociception induced by brief footshock (1 mA, 30 s).

Treatment	Percentage anti-nociception score		5-hydroxytryptamine concentration (ng/g)					
	Non-shock	Shock	Thoracic cord	Pons + medulla	Hypothalamus	Hippocampus	Midbrain	Cortex
Vehicle	107.4 ± 25 (10)	211.9 ± 47.2† (10)	300 ± 30 (9)	336 ± 54 (9)	600 ± 73 (10)	229 ± 65 (8)	576 ± 78 (9)	362 ± 51 (10)
5,7-Dihydroxy-tryptamine	95.7 ± 29.8 (7)	208.6 ± 38.6† (7)	360 ± 32* (7)	257 ± 33** (7)	164 ± 32** (7)	48 ± 19** (7)	253 ± 45** (7)	101 ± 21** (7)
% Change			+20%	−23%	−73%	−79%	−56%	−72%

Values are means ± s.d. Number of rats in brackets. Rats were pretreated with desmethylimipramine (25 mg/kg, i.p.) and injected bilaterally with 4 μg 5,7-dihydroxytryptamine in 0.5 μl vehicle into the medial raphé (coordinates from Konig and Klippell (1963). A, −0.16 mm; L, ± 3.0 mm; H, −8.0 mm from the surface of the skull) at 1 μl/min. Other procedures as Table 6.6. †$p < 0.001$ compared with non-shock controls; *$p < 0.01$, **$p < 0.001$ compared with vehicle-treated rats., (Data from Hutson *et al.*, 1982.)

TABLE 6.8 Effect of *p*-chlorophenylalanine on anti-nociception induced by brief (2 mA, 30 s) or prolonged (2 mA, 30 min) footshock.

		Percentage anti-nociception score (tail-flick method)	
Shock time (min)	Treatment	Non-shock	Shock
0.5	Vehicle	109.6 ± 24.1 (10)	199.9 ± 31.2 (10)*
0.5	*p*-chlorophenylalanine	115.8 ± 21.8 (9)	351.9 ± 125.1 (9)*,††
30	Vehicle	102.9 ± 18.3 (8)	152.3 ± 16.9 (8)*
30	*p*-chlorophenylalanine	104.1 ± 17.1 (8)	111.9 ± 38.5 (8)†

Values are means ± s.d. Number of rats in brackets. Rats were injected with either 0.9% saline or *p*-chlorophenylalanine 150 mg/kg i.p. 72, 48, and 24 h before testing. Percentage score was determined by Procedure 2 for rats shocked for 30 s and by Procedure 3 for rats shocked for 30 min. *$p <$ 0.001 compared with non-shock rats, †$p < 0.02$, †† 0.01 compared with vehicle-treated shocked rats (Student's *t* test). (Data from Tricklebank *et al.*, 1984a.)

TABLE 6.9 Effects of *p*-chloroamphetamine, fenfluramine, and fluoxetine on anti-nociception induced by brief footshock (1m A, 30 s).

Treatment	Percentage anti-nociception score (paw-lick method)	
	Non-shock	Shock
Saline	113.9 ± 27.0 (10)	204.8 ± 52.4** (8)
p-chloroamphetamine (1.5 mg/kg, 30 min before test)	122.0 ± 36.3 (17)	155.3 ± 41.7*,†† (17)
Saline	103.7 ± 33.9 (10)	206.4 ± 48.2** (9)
Fenfluramine (5 mg/kg, 30 min before test)	115.1 ± 32.3 (9)	147.4 ± 23.9†† (9)
Saline	115.5 ± 51.0 (24)	194.7 ± 71.5** (23)
Fluoxetine 10 mg/kg, 120 min before test)	120.9 ± 43.7 (14)	152.1 ± 57.7† (15)

Values are means ± s.d. Number of rats in brackets. Anti-nociception score was determined by Procedure 1. $^{*}p < 0.02$, $^{**}p < 0.001$ compared with non-shocked rats. † $p < 0.05$, ††$p < 0.01$. compared with saline-treated shocked animals. (Data from Tricklebank *et al.*, 1982.)

obtained with fluoxetine, a specific 5-hydroxytryptamine reuptake inhibitor (Fuller and Wong, 1977).

In contrast to Snow *et al.* (1982) who found that quipazine (a 5-hydroxytryptamine agonist) increased and BC105 (a 5-hydroxytryptamine receptor antagonist) decreased anti-nociception induced by brief shock, we found that drugs acting directly on central 5-hydroxytryptamine receptors were on the whole, without effect. Thus several 5-hydroxytryptamine receptor antagonists (Table 6.10) and two potent 5-hydroxytryptamine agonists (Table 6.11) were inactive. However, anti-nociception was attenuated by 5-methoxy-*N,N*-dimethyltryptamine, an agonist that (unlike the other drugs used) is structurally similar to 5-hydroxytryptamine. It is also of interest that this drug has recently been shown to affect the availability of both 5-hydroxytryptamine and dopamine as it inhibits their reuptake and enhances their release in rat brain synaptosomes (Berge *et al.*, 1983). Shock-induced anti-nociception was attenuated by another 5-hydroxytryptamine agonist MK212 but this drug may also affect dopaminergic systems as it has been shown to increase striatal homovanillic acid concentration (Clineschmidt, 1979). Unexpectedly for a 5-hydroxytryptamine agonist, MK212 also antagonizes morphine analgesia and the analgesia induced by the GABA agonist THIP (Murray *et al.*, 1983).

How may the clear effects on shock-induced anti-nociception of drugs which alter 5-hydroxytryptamine availability but the general lack of effect of 5-hydroxytryptamine agonists and antagonists be explained? One possibility is that a hitherto unrecognized 5-hydroxytryptamine receptor is involved. Another possibility is that drugs which alter 5-hydroxytryptamine release influence the analgesia via recognized receptors but that 5-hydroxytryptamine is not involved in the physiological anti-nociceptive effect of brief footshock, i.e. in the effect that occurs in the absence of drugs. Results in Table 6.12 and 6.13 indicate that this may be correct. They show that the attenuation of the anti-nociceptive effect of brief footshock by fenfluramine or 5-methoxy-*N,N*-dimethyltryptamine is prevented by the antagonists cyproheptadine and methiothepin even though the latter drugs have no effect when given alone (Hutson *et al.*, 1983).

How released 5-hydroxytryptamine inhibits the anti-nociceptive effect of brief footshock is not clear. As the analgesia increases with increasing shock intensity (Figure 6.1) it could be that 5-hydroxytryptamine decreases the perceived intensity of the shock. While this possibility cannot be excluded, results in Table 6.14 shows that 5-methoxy-*N,N*-dimethyltryptamine, which is a very rapidly acting 5-hydroxytryptamine agonist, still opposed footshock-induced anti-nociception, as measured by tail-flick, when given after the termination of shock. Since the same dose of the drug did not affect tail-flick latencies in the absence of footshock it did not appear to be acting simply by decreasing basal pain sensitivity. Another possibility is that pharmacologically released 5-hydroxytryptamine may affect the response to brief footshock by

TABLE 6.10 Effect of 5-hydroxytryptamine receptor antagonists on anti-nociception induced by brief footshock (1 mA, 30 s).

Treatment	Percentage anti-nociception score (paw-lick method)	
	Non-shock	Shock
0.9% NaCl	103.0 ± 27.8 (10)	216.8 ± 44.3 (9)**
Cyproheptadine (10 mg/kg, 20 min)	108.6 ± 45.9 (10)	189.5 ± 64.7 (9)*
0.9% NaCl	97.3 ± 19.7 (10)	218.9 ± 48.9 (10)**
Methiothepin (2.5 mg/kg, 30 min)	131.1 ± 52.1 (9)	217.1 ± 68.7 (9)**
Mianserin (2.5 mg/kg, 30 min)	129.3 ± 45.1 (10)	232.7 ± 99.4 (9)**
0.9% NaCl	128.1 ± 38.3 (10)	291.4 ± 88.0 (9)**
Methysergide (2 mg/kg, 120 min)	111.2 ± 38.3 (11)	252.0 ± 88.4 (9)**
0.9% NaCl	97.7 ± 23.4 (10)	220.9 ± 66.2 (9)**
Metergoline (5 mg/kg, 120 min)	108.8 ± 40.0 (9)	255.4 ± 72.1 (10)**
0.9% NaCl	101.3 ± 31.4 (10)	209.2 ± 32.1 (10)**
Metergoline (1 mg/kg, 120 min)	110.0 ± 24.5 (9)	180.8 ± 51.3 (10)**

Values are means ± s.d. Number of rats in brackets. All drugs were given i.p. Percentage anti-nociception score was determined by Procedure 1. *$p < 0.01$, **$p < 0.001$ compared with non-shock controls (Student's t test).

TABLE 6.11 Effects of 5-methoxy-*N,N*-dimethyltryptamine, MK212, trifluoromethylphenylpiperazine and quipazine on anti-nociception induced by brief footshock (1 mA, 30 s).

Treatment	Percentage anti-nociception score (paw-lick method)	
	Non-shock	Shock
0.9% NaCl	103 ± 27.8 (10)	216.8 ± 44.3* (10)
5-methoxy-*N,N*-dimethyltryptamine (2 mg/kg, 20 min before test)	116.2 ± 39.3 (10)	150.8 ± 49.5† (10)
0.9% NaCl	104.5 ± 33.4 (9)	209.5 ± 73.8* (10)
MK212 (2.5 mg/kg, 30 min before test)	111.0 ± 35.3 (8)	130.3 ± 38.2† (11)
0.9% NaCl	128.1 ± 38.3 (10)	291.4 ± 88.0* (10)
Trifluoromethylphenylpiperazine (10 mg/kg, 120 min before test)	113.2 ± 33.7 (9)	267.0 ± 79.2* (10)
0.9% NaCl	97.3 ± 19.7 (10)	219.0 ± 49.0* (10)
Quipazine (2.5 mg/kg, 30 min before test)	117.4 ± 55.1 (10)	225.9 ± 72.7* (10)

Values are means ± s.d. Number of rats in brackets. Percentage anti-nociception score was calculated using Procedure 1. *$p < 0.001$ compared with non-shock animals; † $p < 0.01$ compared with saline-treated shocked rats. (Data from Tricklebank *et al.*, 1982).

TABLE 6.12 Effects of cyproheptadine and methiothepin on the inhibition of shock-induced anti-nociception by fenfluramine.

Treatment		Percentage anti-nociception score (paw-lick method)	
		Non-shock	Shock
Experiment 1			
0.9% NaCl	0.9% NaCl	124.2 ± 24.0	215.6 ± 59.6***
Cyproheptadine	0.9% NaCl	120.9 ± 19.2	198.8 ± 89.3*
0.9% NaCl	Fenfluramine	126.7 ± 19.4	142.6 ± 26.6†
Cyproheptadine	Fenfluramine	130.7 ± 13.8	208.7 ± 42.5***,†
Experiment 2			
0.9% NaCl	0.9% NaCl	113.1 ± 11.2	197.7 ± 29.9***
Methiothepin	0.9% NaCl	119.4 ± 10.5	198.4 ± 35.1***
0.9% NaCl	Fenfluramine	121.0 ± 17.9	150.6 ± 18.8**,††
Methiothepin	Fenfluramine	107.0 ± 13.6	224.6 ± 42.9***,‡

Values are means ± s.d. 10 rats/group. Fenfluramine (5 mg/kg i.p.) was injected 30 min before shock (2 mA, 30 s). Cyproheptadine (10 mg/kg, i.p.) was injected 90 min before shock. Methiothepin (2.5 mg/kg, i.p.) was injected 60 min before shock. Percentage anti-nociception score was determined using Procedure 2. *$p < 0.02$, **$p < 0.01$, ***$p < 0.001$, compared with non-shock controls; † $p < 0.01$, †† $p < 0.001$ compared with shocked rats given 0.9% NaCl only; ‡ $p < 0.001$ compared with shocked rats given 0.9% NaCl and fenfluramine. (Data from Hutson *et al.*, 1983.)

TABLE 6.13 Effects of cyproheptadine and methiothepin on the inhibition of shock-induced anti-nociception by 5-methoxy-N,N-dimethyltryptamine.

Treatment		Percentage anti-nociception score (tail-flick method)	
		Non-shock	Shock
Experiment 1			
0.9% NaCl	0.9% NaCl	122.1 ± 18.2	201.2 ± 53.5**
Cyproheptadine	0.9% NaCl	128.5 ± 16.3	181.2 ± 26.8**
0.9% NaCl	5-methoxy-*N,N*-dimethyltryptamine	131.9 ± 10.3	127.9 ± 13.2 †
Cyproheptadine	5-methoxy-*N,N*-dimethyltryptamine	124.6 ± 13.2	180.9 ± 32.8**††
Experiment 2			
0.9% NaCl	0.9% NaCl	99.7 ± 12.5	183.5 ± 25.9**
Methiothepin	0.9% NaCl	128.7 ± 19.4	164.4 ± 13.2**
0.9% NaCl	5-methoxy-*N,N*-dimethyltryptamine	120.3 ± 18.5	112.5 ± 28.6 †
Methiothepin	5-methoxy-*N,N*-dimethyltryptamine	118.9 ± 20.5	155.9 ± 31.6*,†

Values are means ± s.d. 9/10 rats per group. 5-Methoxy-*N,N*-dimethyltryptamine was injected 1 min before footshock (2 mA/30 s). Other drugs were injected 60 min before shock at the same dose as in Table 6.12. Anti-nociception score was determined by Procedure 2. *$p < 0.01$, **$p < 0.001$ compared with non-shock controls; †$p < 0.001$ compared with shocked rats given 0.9% NaCl only; ‡$p < 0.01$, ‡‡$p < 0.001$ compared with shocked rats given 0.9% NaCl and 5-methoxy-*N,N*-dimethyltryptamine. (Data from Hutson *et al.*, 1983.)

Table 6.14 Effect on anti-nociception of 5-methoxy-*N,N*-dimethyltryptamine given before, after or without footshock (2 mA, 30 s).

Treatment	Percentage anti-nociception score (tail-flick method)		
	Pre-shock	1 min post-shock	2.5 min post-shock
Experiment 1 (shock)			
Group 1. 0.9% NaCl before and after shock	116.9 ± 23.7 (19)	147.9 ± 44.8* (18)	155.1 ± 42.7** (19)
Group 2. 5-methoxy-*N,N*-dimethyltryptamine (1 mg/kg i.p.) before shock; 0.9% NaCl after shock	112.6 ± 33.3 (7)	90.4 ± 29.4† (7)	89.6 ± 41.6† (7)
Group 3. 0.9% NaCl before shock, 5-methoxy-*N,N*-dimethyltryptamine (1 mg/kg i.p.) after shock	125.7 ± 26.9 (22)	158.4 ± 39.1** (21)	116.9 ± 43.2† (22)
Experiment 2 (non-shock)			
0.9% NaCl injections for Group 1	108 ± 20.5 (17)	113.2 ± 27.4 (17)	114.4 ± 30.0 (17)
0.9% NaCl and 5-methoxy-*N,N*-dimethyltryptamine injections as for Group 3	111.9 ± 17.2 (25)	124.4 ± 30.5 (25)	124.5 ± 44.3 (24)

Values are means ± s.d. Number of rats in brackets. Immediately after determining pre-shock latencies (L1 and L2) animals were injected i.p. with either 0.9% NaCl (Experiment 1, Groups 1 and 3) or 5-methoxy-*N,N*-dimethyltryptamine 1 mg/kg (Experiment 1, Group 2). After returning to the home cage for 1 min animals were shocked and immediately injected with either saline (Groups 1 and 2) or 5-methoxy-*N,N*-dimethyltryptamine (Group 3) and returned to the home cage. Tail-flick latency was determined in all animals at 1 and 2.5 min after termination of shock. In a separate experiment the above procedure was repeated as described for Groups 1 and 3 except that animals were not shocked but remained in the home cage for an additional 30 s. Each experiment was done twice and the results combined.
Percentage anti-nociception score was determined by Procedure 2. *$p < 0.02$, **$p < 0.01$ compared with pre-shock controls, †$p < 0.01$ compared with 0.9% NaCl-treated shocked rats using Student's *t* test. (Data from Hutson *et al.*, 1983.)

interfering with memory processes. We have shown (Table 6.2) that anti-nociception due to brief footshock is dependent on exposing the rats to the analgesia test before shock and have tentatively interpreted this as due to the formation of an association between the noxious heat and subsequent footshock so that subsequent tail-flick responses were delayed. Since intracranial injections of 5-hydroxytryptamine (Essman, 1978) or systemic injections of *p*-chloroamphetamine (Archer *et al.*, 1981) cause retrograde amnesia it may be that 5-methoxy-*N,N*-dimethyltryptamine (and by implication 5-hydroxytryptamine) disrupt the association between the noxious heat and brief footshock so that the anti-nociceptive response to the latter is opposed. This mechanism would not be expected to occur following more prolonged footshock as the resultant anti-nociception does not require pre-exposure to the noxious heat (Table 6.2).

DOPAMINE

There have been conflicting reports concerning the involvement of central dopaminergic pathways in pain sensitivity and morphine anti-nociception (Nakamura *et al.*, 1973; Dunai-Kovacs and Szekely, 1977; Gonzalez *et al.*, 1981; Robertson *et al.*, 1981). Similarly, the evidence for dopamine being involved in stress-induced anti-nociception is also conflicting. thus, Kulkarni (1980), Doi and Sawa (1980), and Jensen and Smith (1982a) showed that haloperidol, a dopamine receptor antagonist, attenuated anti-nociception induced by brief footshock, prolonged immobilization, or prolonged tail-shock. In contrast, Snow *et al.* (1982) found that apomorphine, a dopamine receptor agonist, attenuated and haloperidol enhanced anti-nociception induced by brief footshock, while Buckett (1981) found that anti-nociception induced by tail-shock was unaffected by dopaminergic drugs. In agreement with Snow *et al.* (1982), we found that non-cataleptic doses of the antagonists pimozide and haloperidol increased the anti-nociceptive effect of brief footshock (Table 6.15). Furthermore, the specific D_2 agonist LY141865 (Tsurata *et al.*, 1981) but not the specific D_1 agonist SKF38393 (Setler *et al.*, 1978) attenuated the anti-nociceptive response to brief footshock which suggests that D_2 receptors are involved (Table 6.16). Consistent with previous reports of their anti-nociceptive activity in the absence of stress, both apomorphine (Jensen and Smith, 1982b) and amphetamine (Kubota *et al.*, 1982) increased pre-shock paw-lick latencies. Consequently, while these drugs appear to attenuate the anti-nociceptive effect of footshock inasmuch as they decrease the shock-induced increment of latency, the test and control groups are not strictly comparable and consequently the effects of these drugs are not easily interpreted.

The discrepancy between our finding (Tricklebank *et al.*, 1984b) of an inverse relation between dopamine and footshock-induced anti-nociception and the positive relationship found by Doi and Sawa (1980) and Kulkarni (1980) may be

TABLE 6.15 Effects of pimozide and haloperidol on anti-nociception induced by brief footshock (1mA, 30 s).

		Treatment	Latency (s) L1 (pre-shock)	L2 (pre-shock)	L3 (post-shock)
Experiment 1	Tail-flick	Vehicle (10)	3.0 ± 0.39	3.38 ± 0.90	5.92 ± 1.20†
		Pimozide (10)	3.33 ± 0.92	3.66 ± 0.66	6.62 ± 1.05 †
		Haloperidol (10)	2.92 ± 0.30	2.94 ± 0.64	6.82 ± 1.13 †
Experiment 2	Paw-lick	Vehicle (9)	19.5 ± 7.9	20.0 ± 4.7	38.8 ± 7.04 †
		Pimozide (10)	20.6 ± 5.1	21.5 ± 4.4	56.9 ± 15.1**,†
Experiment 3	Paw-lick	Vehicle (10)	22.1 ± 5.3	18.6 ± 2.7	37.6 ± 7.5 †
		Haloperidol (10)	18.7 ± 6.6	16.9 ± 2.7	45.9 ± 9.8*,†

Values are means ± s.d. Number of rats in brackets. Pimozide (1 mg/kg i.p.) and haloperidol (0.2 mg/kg i.p.) were given 60 min before footshock (1 mA, 30 s). $*p < 0.05$, $**p < 0.01$ (t test for independent samples) compared with vehicle-treated rats. $†p < 0.001$ (t test for paired observations) compared with L2 values for same group of rats. (Data from Tricklebank *et al.*, 1984b.)

TABLE 6.16 Effects of dopamine receptor agonists and amphetamine on anti-nociception induced by brief footshock (1 mA, 30 s).

			Latency (s)		
		Treatment	L1 (pre-shock)	L2 (pre-shock)	L3 (post-shock)
Experiment 1	Tail-flick	Vehicle (10)	4.0 ± 0.55	4.48 ± 0.85	6.93 ± 0.83†
		SKF 38393 (10)	4.01 ± 0.58	4.40 ± 0.38	7.02 ± 0.51†
		LY 141865 (10)	4.13 ± 0.40	4.76 ± 0.67	6.12 ± 0.69*,†
Experiment 2	Paw-lick	Vehicle (9)	20.4 ± 6.0	22.7 ± 5.7	42.8 ± 10.8 †
		Apomorphine (10)	38.0 ± 9.6****	36.0 ± 12.8**	48.7 ± 10.1 †
Experiment 3	Paw-lick	Vehicle (9)	22.1 ± 4.0	18.1 ± 3.2	41.6 ± 10.2 †
		Amphetamine (9)	37.8 ± 13.3***	29.5 ± 9.4***	46.7 ± 10.8 †

Values are means ± s.d. Number of rats in brackets. SKF 38393 (2.5 mg/kg, i.p. 60 min). LY 141865 (5 mg/kg, i.p., 60 min). Apomorphine (0.75 mg/kg, s.c., 30 min) and amphetamine (2 mg/kg, i.p. 90 min). $^{*}p < 0.05$, $^{**}p < 0.02$, $^{***}p < 0.01$, $^{****}p < 0.001$ compared with vehicle-treated rats (Student's *t* test for independent groups). $^{\dagger}p < 0.001$ compared with L2 values for same group of rats (Student's *t* test for paired observations). (Data from Tricklebank *et al.*, 1984b.)

Table 6.17 Effect of pimozide on anti-nociception induced by brief (30 s) or prolonged (30 min) footshock (2 mA).

Footshock (min)	Treatment	Tail-flick latency (s)		
		L1 (pre-shock)	L2 (pre-shock)	L3 (post-shock)
0.5	Vehicle (10)	4.03 ± 0.46	4.79 ± 0.73	9.31 ± 1.51
	Pimozide (10)	4.06 ± 0.70	4.26 ± 0.51	11.39 ± 2.28*,††
30	Vehicle (8)	3.82 ± 1.02	4.15 ± 0.75	7.44 ± 2.94
	Pimozide (9)	4.37 ± 0.43	4.60 ± 0.74	5.0 ± 1.1*, †

Values are means ± s.d. Number of rats in brackets. Pimozide (1 mg/kg, i.p.) was given 30 min before determination of post-shock tail-flick latency (L3). *$p \geqslant 0.05$ compared with rats given vehicle (Student's *t* test for independent samples). †$p < 0.02$, ††$p < 0.001$ compared with L2 values for same group of rats (Student's *t* test for paired observations). (Data from Tricklebank *et al.*, 1984b.)

due to the use of different stressors. Table 6.17 shows that the same dose of pimozide increases the anti-nociceptive effect of 0.5 min footshock, but decreases that due to 30 min footshock. This does not explain the finding by Jensen and Smith (1982a) that haloperidol attenuated the anti-nociceptive effect of brief footshock. However, it should be noted that this effect occurred 5 and 10 min after footshock whereas we determined anti-nociception immediately after shock. Since pimozide and haloperidol did not affect latency values measured before the application of shock, the effects we find on shock-induced anti-nociception can hardly be due to a direct action on motor behaviour. Furthermore, it is unlikely that these drugs increase the anti-nociceptive effect of 30 s shock simply by enhancing responsiveness to shock, as this might be expected to result from administration of dopamine releasers, such as amphetamine, rather than dopamine antagonists. However, it is conceivable that the prevention of the anti-nociceptive effect of 30 min shock by pimozide occurs via an attenuation of responsiveness.

CONCLUDING REMARKS

Table 6.18 summarizes our findings. They show that footshock induces an intensity related decrease in responsiveness to noxious thermal stimuli. When footshock is administered for a brief period (i.e. 30 s) the subsequent anti-nociception is unaffected by naloxone, indicating a lack of involvement of endogenous opioids. It appears to be inhibited by dopamine receptor stimulation and by drugs increasing 5-hydroxytryptamine availability. The effects of drugs which increased 5-hydroxytryptamine availability were blocked by 5-hydroxytryptamine antagonists. As the latter drugs were without effect on the anti-nociception induced by shock alone, 5-hydroxytryptamine probably does not play an important part in the physiological anti-nociceptive effect of brief shock even though this can be strikingly altered by pharmacological manipulation of 5-hydroxytryptamine.

TABLE 6.18 Summary of the effects of naloxone, 5-hydroxytryptamine, dopamine, and pre-shock anti-nociception testing on 30 s and 30 min footshock-induced anti-nociception.

	30 s footshock-induced anti-nociception	30 min footshock-induced anti-nociception
Naloxone	No effect	↓
5 -hydroxytryptamine	↓	↑
Dopamine	↓	↑
Dependence on pre-shock anti-nociception testing	Yes	No

As the anti-nociceptive effect of brief shock depended on pre-exposure to nociceptive testing, the animal is responding as if the shock was contingent upon exposure to the previous response latency determination. The effect may thus be analogous to a passive avoidance paradigm and may involve mechanisms of learning and memory. The apparent association formed between noxious heat and footshock was disrupted by 5-methoxy-*N,N*-dimethyltryptamine (a rapidly acting 5-hydroxytryptamine agonist) when given after the termination of shock. This is consistent with previous reports of memory processes being disrupted by 5-hydroxytryptamine.

Following prolonged (i.e. 30 min) footshock at the same intensity as that used in the experiments on brief footshock, dependence on pre-shock exposure to nociceptive testing was no longer apparent. This could be due to the association not being retained for 30 min or to a disruption of the association by prolonged shock. In striking contrast with the results obtained when shock was applied for 30 s, the anti-nociception was attenuated by naloxone, by the dopamine receptor antagonist pimozide, and the tryptophan hydroxylase inhibitor *p*-chlorophenylalanine.

In view of the completely different characteristics of the anti-nociception following brief and prolonged shock it seems hardly surprising that the literature on stress-induced anti-nociception contains numerous discrepancies. These observations and the finding that the anti-nociceptive effect of brief shock depended on pre-exposure to the anti-nociception test emphasize the crucial importance of experimental design in this field of research (see Chapter 8).

REFERENCES

Amir, S., and Amit, Z. (1979). Enhanced analgesic effects of stress following chronic administration of naltrexone in rats. *Eur., J. Pharmacol.*, **59**, 137–140.

Archer, T., Ogren, S. O., and Johansson, C. (1981). The acute effect of *p*-chloroamphetamine on the retention of fear conditioning in the rat: evidence for a role of serotonin in memory consolidation. *Neurosci. Lett.*, **25**, 75–81.

Berge, O.-G., Chacho, D., and Hole, K. (1983). Inhibitory effect of 5-methoxy-*N,N*-dimethyltryptamine on the synaptosomal uptake of 5-hydroxytryptamine. *Eur. J. Pharmacol.*, **90**, 293–296.

Bhattacharya, S. K., Keshary, P. R., and Sanyal, A. K. (1978). Immobilization stress-induced antinociception in rats: possible role of serotonin and prostaglandins. *Eur. J. Pharmacol.*, **50**, 83–85.

Bodnar, R. J., Kelly, D. D., Spiaggia, A., Ehrenberg, C., and Glusman, M. (1978a). Dose-dependent reductions by naloxone of analgesia induced by cold-water stress. *Pharmacol. Biochem. and Behav.*, **8**. 667–672.

Bodnar, R. J., Kelly, D. D., Steiner, S. S., and Glusman, M. (1978b). Stress produced analgesia and morphine-produced analgesia: lack of cross tolerance. *Pharmacol. Biochem. and Behav.*, **8**, 661–666.

Bodnar, R. J., Kelly, D. D., and Glusman, M. (1979). 2-deoxy-D-glucose analgesia: influences of opiate and non-opiate factors. *Pharmacol. Biochem. and Behav.*, **11**, 297–301.

Buckett, W. R. (1979). Peripheral stimulation in mice induces short duration analgesia preventable by naloxone. *Eur. J. Pharmacol.,* **58**, 169–178.

Buckett, W. R. (1981). Pharmacological studies on stimulation-produced analgesia in mice. *Eur. J. Pharmacol.,* **69**, 281–290.

Chance, W. T., and Rosecrans, J. A. (1979a). Lack of effect of naloxone on autoanalgesia. *Pharmacol. Biochem. and Behav.,* **11**, 643–646.

Chance, W. T., and Rosecrans, J. A. (1979b). Lack of cross-tolerance between morphine and autoanalgesia. *Pharmacol. Biochem. and Behav.,* **11**, 639–642.

Chance, W. T., and Schechter, M. D. (1979). Autoanalgesia: blockade by yohimbine. *Eur. J. Pharmac.,* **58**, 89–90.

Chance, W. T., White, A. C., Krynock, G. M., and Rosecrans, J. A. (1977). Autoanalgesia: behaviourally activated antinociception. *Eur. J. Pharmacol.,* **44**, 283–284.

Chesher, G. B., and Chan, B. (1977). Footshock induced analgesia in mice: its reversal by naloxone and cross tolerance with morphine. *Life Sci.,* **21**, 1569–1574.

Clineschmidt, B. V. (1979). MK212: A serotonin like agonist in the CNS. *Gen. Pharmac.,* **10**, 287–290.

Curzon, G., and Green, A. R. (1970). Rapid method for the determination of 5-hydroxytryptamine and 5-hydroxyindoleacetic acid in small regions of rat brain. *Br. J. Pharmac.,* **39**, 653–655.

Curzon, G., Kantamaneni, B. D., and Tricklebank, M. D. (1981). A comparison of an improved *o*-phthaladehyde method and high pressure liquid chromatography in the determination of brain 5-hydroxyindoles of rats treated with L-tryptophan and *p*-chlorophenylalanine. *Br. J. Pharmac.,* **73**, 555–562.

D'Amour, F. E., and Smith, D. L. (1941). A method of determining loss of pain sensation. *J. Pharm. Exp. Ther.,* **72**, 74–79.

Doi, T., and Sawa, N. (1980). Antagonistic effects of psycholeptic drugs on stress induced analgesia. *Arch. Int. Pharmacodyn.,* **247**, 264–274.

Dunai-Kovacs, Z., and Szekely, J. I. (1977). Effect of apomorphine on the antinociceptive activity of morphine. *Psychopharmacology,* **53**, 65–72.

Essman, W. B. (1978). Serotonin in learning and memory, in *Serotonin in Health and Disease, Vol. 3, The Central Nervous System* (ed. W. B. Essman), Spectrum New York, pp. 69–143.

Frederickson, R. C. A., Burgis, V., and Edwards, J. D. (1977). Hyperalgesia induced by naloxone follows diurnal rhythm in responsivity to painful stimuli. *Science,* **198**, 756–758.

Fuller, R. L., and Wong, D. T. (1977). Inhibition of serotonin reuptake. *Fedn. Proc. Fedn. Am. Socs. Exp. Biol.,* **36**, 2154–2158.

Gonzalez, J. P., Sewell, R. D. E., and Spencer, P. S. J. (1981). Dopaminergic involvement in the hyperalgesic effect of nomifensine. *Life Sci.,* **28**, 951–956.

Grau, J. W., Hyson, R. L., Maier, S. F., Madden, IV, J., and Barchas, J. D. (1981). Long-term stress-induced analgesia and activation of the opiate system. *Science,* **213**, 1409–1411.

Hayes, R. L., Bennett, G. J., Newlon, P. G., and Mayer, D. J. (1978). Behavioural and physiological studies of non-narcotic analgesia in the rat elicited by certain environmental stimuli. *Brain Res.,* **155**, 69–90.

Hutson, P. H., Tricklebank, M. D., and Curzon, G. (1982). Enhancement of footshock induced analgesia by spinal 5,7-dihydroxytryptamine lesions. *Brain Res.,* **237**, 367–372.

Hutson, P. H., Tricklebank, M. D., and Curzon, G. (1983). Analgesia induced by brief footshock: blockade by fenfluramine and 5-methoxy-*N,N*-dimethyltryptamine and prevention of blockade by 5HTantagonists. *Brain Res.,* **279**, 105–110.

Jensen, T. S., and Smith, D. F. (1982a). Monoaminergic mechanisms in stress induced analgesia. *J. Neural Trans.*, **53**, 247–255.
Jensen, T. S., and Smith, D. F. (1982b). Dopaminergic effects on tail-flick response in spinal rats. *Eur. J. Pharmacol.*, **79**, 129–133.
Konig, J. F. R., and Klippell, R. A. (1963). *The Rat Brain. A Stereotaxic Atlas*. Williams & Wilkins, Baltimore.
Kubota, K., Matsuoka, Y., Sakuma, M., Satoh, S.-I, Urono, T., and Sunagane, N. (1982). Characteristic of analgesia induced by non-catecholic phenylethylamines in mice. *Life Sci.*, **31**, 1221–1224.
Kulkarni, S. K. (1980). Heat and other physiological stress-induced analgesia: catecholamine mediated and naloxone reversible response. *Life Sci.*, **27**, 185–188.
Lai, Y.-Y., and Chan, S. H. H. (1981). Shortened pain response time following repeated algesiometric tests in rats. *Physiol. and Behav.*, **28**, 1111–1113.
Lewis, J. W., Cannon, J. T., and Liebeskind, J. C. (1980). Opioid and nonopioid mechanisms of stress analgesia. *Science*, **208**, 623–625.
Lewis, J. W., Sherman, J. E., and Liebeskind, J. C. (1981). Opioid and nonopioid stress analgesia: assessment of tolerance and cross tolerance with morphine. *J. Neurosci.*, **1**, 358–363.
Madden, IV, J., Akil, H., Patrick, R. L., and Barchas, J. D. (1977). Stress induced parallel changes in central opioid levels and pain responsiveness in the rat. *Nature*, **265**, 358–360.
Maier, S. F., Davies, S., Grau, J. W., Jackson, R. L., Morrison, D. H., Moye, T., Madden, IV, J., and Barchas, J. D. (1980). Opiate antagonists and long term analgesic reaction induced by inescapable shock in rats. *J. Comp. Physiol. Psychol.*, **94**, 1172–1183.
Messing, R. B., Fisher, L. A., Phebus, L., and Lytle, L. D. (1976). Interaction of diet and drugs in the regulation of brain 5-hydroxyindoles and the response to painful electric shock. *Life Sci.*, **18**, 707–714.
Murray, T. F., McGill, W., and Cheney, D. L. (1983). A comparison of the analgesic properties of 4,5,6,7-tetrahydroisoxazolo[5,4,-c]pyridin-3-ol (THIP) and 6-chloro-2[I-piperazinyl]pyrazine (MK212). *Europ. J. Pharmacol.*, **90**, 179–184.
Nakamura, K. R., Kuntzmann, A., Maggio, J., and Conney, A. M. (1973). Decrease in morphines analgesic action and increase in cataleptic action by 6-hydroxydopamine injected bilaterally into caudate and putamen areas. *Neuropharmac.*, **12**, 1153–1158.
Ogren, S.-O., and Holm, A.-C. (1980). Test-specific effects of the 5HT reuptake inhibitors alaproclate and zimelidine on pain sensitivity and morphine analgesia. *J. Neural Trans.*, **47**, 253–271.
Oliverio, A., and Castellano, C. (1982). Classical conditioning of stress induced analgesia. *Physiol. and Behav.*, **25**, 171–172.
Pellegrino, L. J., Pellegrino, A. S., and Cushman, A. J. (1979). *A Stereotaxic Atlas of the Rat Brain*. 2nd ed., Plenum Press, New York.
Puglisi-Allegra, S., Castellano, C., and Oliverio, A. (1982). Circadian variation in stress induced analgesia. *Brain Res.*, **252**, 373–376.
Riffee, W. H., Wilcox, R. E., and Smith, R. V. (1979). Modification of drug induced behavioural arousal by pre-injection routines in mice. *Psychopharm.*, **63**, 1–5.
Robertson, J., Weston, R., Lewis, M. J., and Barasi, S. (1981). Evidence for the potentiation of the antinociceptive action of morphine by bromocriptine. *Neuropharmac.*, **20**, 1029–1032.
Rodgers, R. J., and Deacon, R. M. J. (1981). Footshock-analgesia: prevention by behavioural manipulation but not by naloxone. *Physiol. and Behav.*, **26**, 183–187.

Schlosberg, A. J., and Harvey, J. A. (1978). Diurnal changes in serotonin content of frontal pole and pain sensitivity in the rat. *Physiol. and Behav.*, **20**, 117–120.

Setler, P. E., Sarau, H. M., Zerkle, C. L., and Saunders, H. L. (1978). The central effects of a novel dopamine agonist. *Eur. J. Pharmacol.*, **50**, 419–431.

Shimizu, T., Koja, T., Fujisaki, T., and Fukuda, T. (1981). Effects of methysergide and naloxone on analgesia induced by the peripheral electric stimulation in mice. *Brain Res.*, **208**, 463–467.

Snow, A. E., Tucker, S. M., and Dewey, W. L. (1982). The role of neurotransmitters in stress induced antinociception (SIA). *Pharmacol. Biochem. and Behav.*, **16**, 47–50.

Tenen, S. S. (1967). The effects of *p*-chlorophenylalanine a serotonin depletor on avoidance acquisition, pain sensitivity and behaviour in the rat. *Psychopharmacologia Berlin,* **10**, 204–219.

Terman, G. W., Lewis, J. W., and Liebeskind, J. C. (1982). Role of biogenic amines in stress analgesia. *Proc. West Pharmacol. Soc.*, **25**, 7–10.

Tricklebank, M. D., Hutson, P. H., and Curzon, G. (1982). Analgesia induced by brief footshock is inhibited by 5-hydroxytryptamine but unaffected by antagonists of 5-hydroxytryptamine or by naloxone. *Neuropharmacol.*, **21**, 51–56.

Tricklebank, M. D., Hutson, P. H., and Curzon, G. (1984a). Analgesia induced by brief or more prolonged stress differs in its dependency on naloxone, 5-hydroxytryptamine and previous analgesia testing. *Neuropharmacol.*, **23**, 417–421.

Tricklebank, M. D., Hutson, P. H., and Curzon, G. (1984b). Involvement of dopamine in the antinociceptive response to footshock *Psychopharmacology*, **82**, 185–188.

Trulson, M. E., and Jacobs, B. L. (1976). Behavioural evidence for the rapid release of CNS serotonin by PCA and fenfluramine. *Eur. J. Pharmacol.*, **36**, 149–154.

Tsurata, K., Frey, E. A., Grewe, C. W., Cote, T. E., Eskay, R. L., and Kebabian, J. W. (1981). Evidence that LY 141865 specifically stimulates the D_2 dopamine receptor. *Nature,* **292**, 463–465.

Watkins, L. R., Cobelli, D. A., Faris, P., Aceto, M. D., and Mayer, D. J. (1982). Opiate vs non-opiate footshock induced analgesia (FSIA): the body region shocked is a critical factor. *Brain Res.*, **242**, 299–308.

Wesche, D. L., and Frederickson, R. C. A. (1979). Diurnal differences in opioid peptide levels correlated with nociceptive sensitivity. *Life Sci.*, **24**, 1861–1868.

Yaksh, T. L., and Wilson, P. R. (1979). Spinal serotonin terminal system mediates antinociception. *J. Pharmac. Exp. Ther.*, **208**, 446–453.

Stress-induced Analgesia
Edited by M. D. Tricklebank and G. Curzon

CHAPTER 7

Stress-induced analgesia and avoidance behaviour: possible interactions with serotonergic neurotransmission

S.-O. OGREN, T. ARCHER, and C. JOHANSSON

INTRODUCTION

There is now considerable evidence that various environmental stimuli can activate pain modulatory systems in the brain leading to subsequent changes in behaviour (Watkins and Mayer, 1982). Several stress-inducing interventions including immobilization, tail-shock, or footshock are reported to decrease the unconditioned responsiveness to various noxious stimuli (Madden, 1977; Hayes *et al.*, 1978a; Buckett, 1981). Reduced responsiveness to heat is a consistent finding following inescapable footshock or tail-shock which presumably results in a stress-reaction. Both opioid and non-opioid mechanisms have been implicated in this form of analgesia (Chance, 1980; Lewis *et al.*, 1980). It has been suggested that stress-induced analgesia is mainly due to modification of the affective component of pain since restraint-stress, e.g. immobilization has been found to increase escape latencies but not to affect the latency to paw-lick as measured by a hot-plate method (Amir and Amit, 1979). Exposure to inescapable shock treatment has also been shown to result in performance deficits in active escape reactions from footshock in rats and mice (Weiss *et al.*, 1975; Anisman *et al.*, 1979). However, it is not yet clear whether the escape deficits are due to alterations in the ability to maintain responding or to changes in the perceptive or affective component of pain (Blair *et al.*, 1982). Nevertheless, it should be noted that deficits in shuttle-box active escape responding have only been observed when the animals have received prolonged shock-exposure, e.g. 60 inescapable 6 s shock presentations at 60 s intervals prior to testing (Anisman *et al.*, 1979).

AVOIDANCE AND SHOCK-INDUCED ANALGESIA; METHODOLOGICAL ASPECTS

The exposure of rats to aversive stimuli, such as electric shock also has profound effects on a variety of learned behaviours. Shock will either increase or decrease behavioural output depending on whether its presentation is contingent upon the presence or the absence of specific responses. Animals will generally postpone or decrease responding if a response results in the delivery of signalled or unsignalled shock (punishment) or they will increase frequency of behaviours which result in the escape or avoidance of the delivery of shock (escape or avoidance). In the early two-factor theory of avoidance conditioning it was assumed that exposure to shock or pain resulted in a state of fear which led to a classically conditioned fear response composed of sympathetic autonomic reactions. The avoidance response was mediated via instrumental responses resulting in a reduction of the conditioned fear-reaction by removing the subject from fear-evoking stimuli (Mowrer, 1947). Later theories have emphasized that sympathetic and other physiological responses are not mediators of the avoidance response but are rather indications of unspecified CNS events which may underlie avoidance behaviour (Rescorla and Solomon, 1967).

There are important methodological differences between the presentation of footshock in an avoidance/escape shock paradigm and in paradigms which produce shock-induced analgesia (for summary, see Table 7.1). The major difference is the contingency under which shock is delivered and the conditions under which the behavioural performance is assessed (see Table 7.1). In stress-induced analgesia, shock is mostly administered in one location and the behavioural performance is examined in a different location using a different stimulus (usually radiant heat) to assess the behavioural performance. Moreover, in an active avoidance paradigm, shock is always escapable and is usually signalled. Signalled shock results in a superior performance compared to unsignalled shock. However, it must be emphasized that conditioning

TABLE 7.1 Methodological differences between the shock-induced analgesia and active avoidance paradigms.

Parameters	Shock-induced analgesia	Active avoidance
Shock-type	Inescapable Non-signalled	Escapable or avoidable Signalled
Shock-exposure	Prolonged and continuous	Brief and intermittent
Location of shock-exposure	Mostly different from testing	The same in training and in testing

factors can also be important in shock-induced analgesia. Thus, rats trained to associate environmental cues with shock-presentation in a classical conditioning paradigm were found to acquire a conditioned analgesia (Chance *et al.*, 1979; Watkins and Mayer, 1982). Thus, both in avoidance and in shock-induced analgesia paradigms, fear-conditioning can occur to the warning stimulus or to other components of the test situation present at conditioning and the learned fear response appears under certain circumstances to result in some degree of decreased response to the pain-provoking stimulus (Chance *et al.*, 1979; Watkins and Mayer, 1982).

There is now considerable evidence that central serotonergic neurones are important in aversive learning processes (Essman, 1973; Ogren *et al.*, 1981; Ogren, 1982a) and in shock-induced analgesia (Curzon *et al.*, 1980, 1981; Tricklebank *et al.*, 1982). Because of the possible involvement of 5HT in aversive learning and in nociception it was of interest to determine whether alterations in 5HT neurotransmission result in parallel changes in active avoidance and in nociceptive responding. In addition, a fear-retention paradigm was used to examine the involvement of 5HT in shock-induced analgesia and in fear retention (Archer *et al.*, 1981).

SEROTONIN DEPLETION; EFFECTS ON AVOIDANCE AND NOCICEPTIVE PROCESSES

Experimental methods

There is a growing body of experimental data based on protocols involving 5HT depletion implicating central serotonergic (5HT) neurones in a wide range of aversive learning and memory processes (Lorens, 1978; Ogren, 1982a) and in nociceptive processes (Lorens, 1978). Results from different procedures including (1) electrolytic lesions of the 5HT raphé nuclei in the midbrain, (2) administration of the tryptophan hydroxylase inhibitor *p*-chlorophenylalanine, (3) administration of the serotonergic neurotoxin *p*-chloroamphetamine, and (4) intracerebral administration of the 5HT neurotoxins 5,6 and 5,7-dihydroxytryptamine, have shown that manipulation of ascending and/or descending 5HT neurotransmission can affect both the acquisition and retention of aversive learning. In the present chapter, data obtained by the use of *p*-chlorophenylalanine or *p*-chloroamphetamine will mainly be reviewed.

Interpretation of the effects of systemic *p*-chlorophenylalanine treatment is complicated since 5HT is reduced throughout the body, e.g. forebrain regions, the spinal cord and peripheral 5HT stores (Vogt, 1974; Ogren *et al.*, 1980). The behavioural importance of extracerebral 5HT is unknown though it may be relevant that there is evidence of extracerebral mediation of the effect of its precursor tryptophan on motor activity (Tricklebank *et al.*, 1980). A further disadvantage of *p*-chlorophenylalanine is that it causes slight but consistent decreases of brain catecholamine concentrations (Koe and Weissman, 1966).

Another approach to the study of 5HT involvement is by systemic administration of the neurotoxin *p*-chloroamphetamine (Sanders-Bush and Steranka, 1978). This drug produces only minor and transient changes in brain catecholamine neurones and does not deplete peripheral 5HT stores. The long-term effect of a single dose of *p*-chloroamphetamine develops within three days and is clearly distinguished from its acute 5HT releasing action (see below). These long-term effects seem mainly to involve the ascending 5HT pathways originating from the B7–B9 group with marginal effects on the descending 5HT pathways (Köhler *et al.*, 1978). An advantage of the use of *p*-chloroamphetamine is that its neurotoxic action can be blocked by inhibitors of the neuronal uptake of 5HT such as zimelidine.

EFFECTS OF *p*-CHLOROPHENYLALANINE AND LONG TERM *p*-CHLOROAMPHETAMINE ON AVOIDANCE AND NOCICEPTION

Recent studies have indicated that the effects of 5HT depletion on both nociception and avoidance depend upon the test situation used (Lorens, 1978; Ogren *et al.*, 1981). Table 7.2 summarizes the reported effects of *p*-chlorophenylalanine and *p*-chloroamphetamine. In most studies, *p*-chlorophenylalanine increases the responsiveness of rats to electrical shock whether measured by the jump or flinch threshold, but does not reliably change nociceptive threshold as measured in the hot-plate or tail-flick tests (Harvey *et al.*, 1974; Berge *et al.*, 1983). Thus, these data tend to confirm that brain 5HT depletion by this drug may increase reactivity to certain stimuli including footshock (Tenen, 1967; Fibiger *et al.*, 1972). Long-term *p*-chloroamphetamine on the other hand, appears not to lower flinch threshold but has recently been

Table 7.2 The effects of brain serotonin depletion induced by *p-chlorophenylalanine* (PCPA) and long-term *p-chloroamphetamine* (PCA) (2 × 10 mg/kg) treatment on responses to noxious stimulation and on active avoidance learning in the rat.

		Nociceptive tests		Active avoidance	
Treatment	Flinch-/jump thresholds	Hot-plate	Tail flick	One-way	Two-way
PCPA	↓	0	0	↑,0	↑,0
PCA (2 × 10 mg/kg)	↓ (flinch, 0 = jump	0	0	0	0

The results from nociceptive testing are taken from Berge *et al.*, 1982; and avoidance data are from Ogren *et al.*, 1981; Ogren, 1982a.

reported to lower jump threshold (Berge *et al.*, 1982). In view of the different actions of these drugs on brain 5HT neurones the general increase in reactivity to electrical shock following *p*-chlorophenylalanine administration has been suggested to depend on depletion in the descending 5HT pathways (Berge *et al.*, 1982). Thus, these and related data question the presence of tonic anti-nociceptive activity of the ascending 5HT neurones, while there is considerable evidence for a tonic inhibitory role of the descending 5HT pathways (Yaksh, 1979; Berge, 1982).

Recent observations suggest that aversive stimulation can affect spinal 5HT activity (Yaksh, 1979). Thus, the activation of descending raphé spinal pathways by footshock in the avoidance situation could change the processing of nociceptive information and influence the unconditioned responsiveness to shock and possibly modify subsequent performance (see Watkins and Mayer, 1982). However, there is no evidence of a simple or linear relationship between effects on nociception and avoidance performance. Early studies with *p*-chlorophenylalanine reported enhanced acquisition of a signalled one-way avoidance response (jumping to a platform) when a low footshock intensity was used (Tenen, 1967). Since the drug also decreased jump-threshold it was suggested that the enhanced rate of acquisition probably was due to the enhanced reactivity to shock (Tenen, 1967). Later studies indicated that this enhancement of avoidance acquisition may depend on both the avoidance situation and shock level (Tenen, 1967; Ogren *et al.*, 1981; Ogren, 1982a). For instance, facilitation of a two-way shuttle avoidance response was not observed following *p*-chlorophenylalanine treatment (Köhler and Lorens, 1978). Such data illustrate that 5HT does not alter avoidance performance merely by altering reflex responses to noxious stimuli.

Since most previous studies were performed under different stimulus conditions we decided to re-examine the effects of long-term *p*-chloroamphetamine and *p*-chlorophenylalanine treatments on both one- and two-way avoidance. Since avoidance learning is aversively motivated and depends on several variables including (1) the general level of unconditioned responsiveness to shock or other stimuli and (2) the intensity of footshock or other stimuli, it was of interest to study active-avoidance acquisition as a function of the unconditioned shock level. Previous data have shown that in the signalled two-way active avoidance situation, strong as opposed to weak shock results in a low rate of acquisition while in the one-way task there is evidence for a linear relationship between shock level and avoidance performance (Moyer and Korn, 1966; McAllister and McAllister, 1971). The lower avoidance rate at high shock levels in the two-way task has been attributed to increased freezing and induction of immobility. If changes in nociceptive threshold bear a direct relationship to avoidance performance, then *p*-chlorophenylalanine treatment (which lowers flinch threshold) should facilitate one-way avoidance at all shock-levels while two-way performance would be facilitated at low and retarded at high shock-levels.

In this study, four treatments were administered as follows: groups of eight rats received *p*-chlorophenylalanine (200, 100 and 100 mg/kg 72, 48, and 24 h respectively before avoidance acquisition), or *p*-chloroamphetamine (2 × 10 mg/kg i.p.), or zimelidine (2 × 20 mg/kg) + *p*-chloroamphetamine (2 × 10 mg/kg) or saline. Pretreatment with zimelidine at this dose blocks the *p*-chloroamphetamine-induced degeneration of 5HT neurones in most terminal regions (Köhler *et al.*, 1978). The drug treatments were administered on two consecutive days, 8 and 7 days before the rats were tested for avoidance acquisition. A separate group of rats received a similar treatment and in addition four escapable shocks (1.0 mA) separated by intervals of 45 s were administered in the avoidance box 24 h prior to acquisition. This treatment is strong enough to produce fear-acquisition and a slight shock induced analgesia (see below). The shock levels in both one-way and two-way conditions were 0.75, 1.5, or 3.0 mA. In the one-way task, *p*-chlorophenylalanine treatment tended to impair avoidance performance at both the low and high shock levels although there was evidence of enhanced acquisition in the middle-range shock level (to be published). However, after *p*-chloroamphetamine treatment, there was no evidence of facilitation at any of the shock levels used. As shown in Figure 7.1, two-way avoidance performance was highly dependent on the shock level. A high shock level tended to impair the avoidance performance in agreement with previous data. Contrary to the prediction that enhanced reactivity to shock would be advantageous at lower shock levels, the *p*-chlorophenylalanine treated rats demonstrated low avoidance performance at both the low and high shock intensities and showed facilitation when 1.5 mA was given. *p*-Chloroamphetamine treated rats on the other hand tended to be impaired at the high shock level but not at the lowest shock level (0.75 mA).

The results obtained on rats pre-exposed to escapable shock are shown in Figure 7.2. It is notable that in the two-way avoidance situation this causes a severe avoidance deficit (compared to results on non-shocked rats). Again, the shock level critically determines the avoidance performance. Thus *p*-chlorophenylalanine causes low avoidance performance at 0.75 mA but facilitates it at 1.5 mA and 3.0 mA while *p*-chloroamphetamine (2 × 10 mg/kg) causes impairment at 1.5 mA but facilitation at 0.75 mA.

These findings demonstrate that shock level has striking effects on two-way avoidance learning in animals depleted of brain 5HT. However, the results are not consistent with the previous prediction of the relationship between avoidance performance and nociception. Moreover, data from non-preshocked rats show that *p*-chlorophenylalanine and *p*-chloroamphetamine treatments which block shock-induced analgesia (see below), do not produce similar effects, indicating different roles of different serotonergic pathways. Moreover, the effects of 5HT depletion and shock level appear to show an interaction in the animals which have been subjected to fear conditioning (shock presentation) prior to the actual acquisition trials.

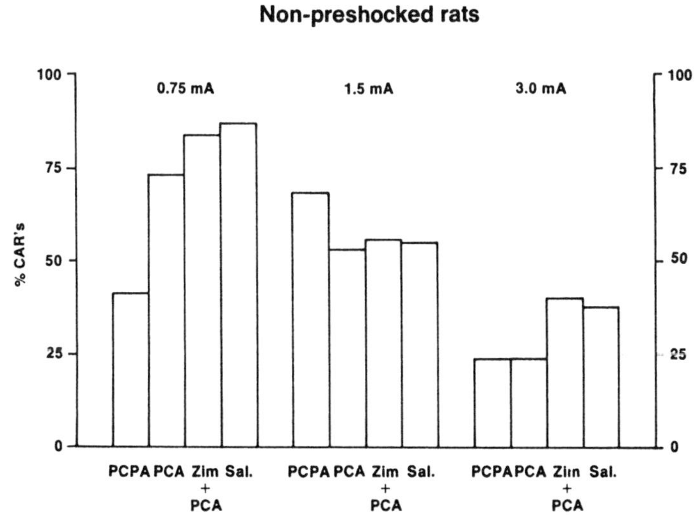

FIGURE **7.1** Effects of brain serotonin depletion on signalled two-way active avoidance acquisition by non-preshocked rats. Brain serotonin was depleted by *p*-chlorophenylalanine (PCPA) and by *p*-chloroamphetamine (PCA) injected at a dose of 10 mg/kg on two consecutive days, 8 and 7 days prior to acquisition. Details of treatment are described in the text. Zimelidine (ZIM/20 mg/kg) was injected prior to each PCA injection (10 mg/kg). The mean conditioned avoidances (CARs) of eight rats are shown. PCPA differed significantly from saline controls at the 0.75 and 3.0 mA.

However, it is notable that *p*-chlorophenylalanine which clearly blocks shock-induced analgesia tended to facilitate avoidance learning at 1.5 and 3.0 mA in preshocked rats. Taken together, results show that central 5HT systems appear to modulate mechanisms involving integration of nociceptive processing in the avoidance learning situation. However, the mechanisms underlying the processing of nociceptive inputs and the conditioning mechanisms seem not to be subserved by identical systems. A particularly interesting observation is that 5HT depletion under certain conditions seems to attenuate the effects of shock pretreatment while in other situations it seems to enhance them (see below).

EFFECTS OF INCREASED 5HT RECEPTOR ACTIVITY ON AVOIDANCE AND NOCICEPTIVE PROCESSES

Experimental methods

In these studies, the acute release of 5HT by *p*-chloroamphetamine was used to examine the effects of increased 5HT receptor activation. The drug when given

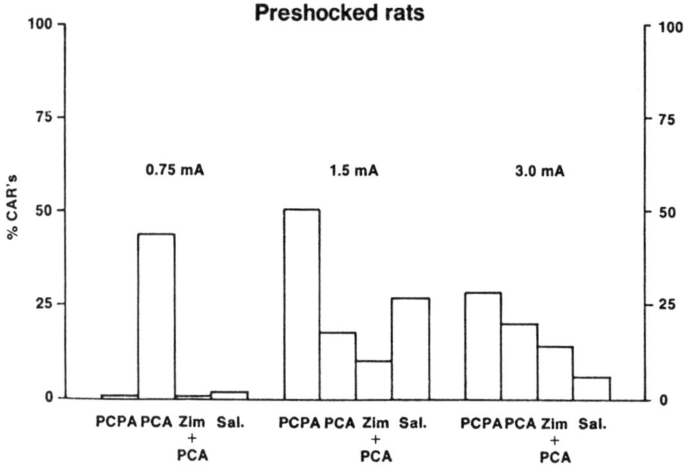

FIGURE 7.2 Effects of brain serotonin depletion on signalled two-way active avoidance acquisition by preshocked rats. For treatment details, see Figure 7.1 legend. Each rat was exposed to four escapable shocks (1.0 mA) 24 h prior to the onset of 100-trial avoidance session. With this exception, identical conditions to those above were maintained.

in low doses rapidly releases serotonin, resulting in an increased concentration at receptor sites (Ogren *et al.*, 1977; Sanders–Bush and Steranka, 1978; Marsden *et al.*, 1979). The selective involvement of 5HT either pre- or post-synaptically can be examined by a variety of pharmacological approaches including prevention of the neuronal uptake of the releasing agent (Ross, 1976), administration of receptor blockers, or prior depletion of the transmitter content (Ogren, 1982b). Both behavioural and biochemical data suggest that the 5HT releasing effect of *p*-chloroamphetamine is blocked by specific inhibitors of neuronal 5HT uptake but not by specific inhibitors of NA uptake (Ross 1975; Ogren *et al.*, 1977). Thus, the drug must be taken up into presynaptic 5HT neurones and then release endogenously stored 5HT to exert its effect.

Effects on nociception and avoidance

Procedures which increase intra-synaptic 5HT and presumably 5HT receptor activity in the brain can moderately increase responses to nociceptive stimulation. Thus, small elevations in hot-plate or tail-flick thresholds have been found following 5HT reuptake inhibition (Ogren and Holm, 1980) or injection of 5HT into the cerebral ventricles (Sewell and Spencer, 1975). However, previous studies have demonstrated that *p*-chloroamphetamine can induce reliable and marked analgesia as measured by the paw compression

(Görlitz and Frey, 1972) and the hot-plate test (Ogren and Holm, 1980). In a recent study, this analgesia was demonstrated with the hot-plate and flinch-jump methods but not with the tail-flick test (Ogren and Berge, 1984). The analgesia was attenuated or blocked by 5HT uptake inhibitors, by 5HT depleters and by lesioning of 5HT terminals. These results indicate that it is mediated via 5HT release.

Several studies have shown that injecting *p*-chloroamphetamine 30 min prior to testing also produces a dose-related inhibition of active avoidance acquisition and retention (Ogren, 1982a, b). Recent observations suggest that a loss in pain-sensitivity, induction of freezing behaviour or loss of locomotor capacities are not a likely cause of the avoidance deficit (Ogren and Johansson, 1984). In addition, the possible relationship between effects of 5HT release on nociception and on avoidance learning has been studied in several recent experiments. To examine the importance of 5HT release for the action of *p*-chloroamphetamine, rats were pretreated with zimelidine (10 mg/kg), a selective 5HT uptake inhibitor, or with desipramine (5 mg/kg), a selective NA uptake inhibitor, prior to injection of *p*-chloroamphetamine (2.5 mg/kg). Zimelidine (but not desipramine) pretreatment completely blocked the impairment of avoidance learning (Ogren, 1982b) and the hot-plate analgesia (Ogren and Berge, 1984) normally induced by *p*-chloroamphetamine (see Figure 7.3). These data indicate that both effects are dependent upon 5HT release.

This conclusion is further supported by the attenuation of both the *p*-chloroamphetamine-induced analgesia and the avoidance deficit by prior depletion of neuronal 5HT by the 5HT synthesis inhibitor *p*-chlorophenylalanine (Ogren and Berge, 1984). It is of particular interest that metergoline failed to block *p*-chloroamphetamine-induced analgesia but markedly blocked the corresponding avoidance deficit (Figure 7.4). Metergoline has been shown to be a 5HT receptor antagonist both in electrophysiological (Sastry and Phillis, 1977) and in behavioural studies (Fuxe *et al.*, 1978) and it is also a potent blocker of both 5-HT_1 and 5-HT_2 receptors (Fuxe *et al.*, 1978; Peroutka *et al.*, 1981). The compound has also been shown to produce hyperalgesia in the hot-plate situation (Ogren and Berge, 1984) suggesting that it blocks 5HT terminals involved in tonic inhibition of nociception. It is therefore likely that the avoidance deficit and the analgesia induced by *p*-chloroamphetamine are both mediated by 5HT release but due to different 5HT dependent mechanisms.

In this context it is notable that a 2.5 mg/kg dose of *p*-chloroamphetamine 60 min after injection produced regional changes in the 5HT levels preferentially in the forebrain region with significant reductions in the cerebral cortex, hippocampus, and striatum while only marginal effects were observed in the hypothalamus and spinal cord (Ogren, 1982b). In view of the possible existence of different 5HT receptor types in the brain and spinal cord with

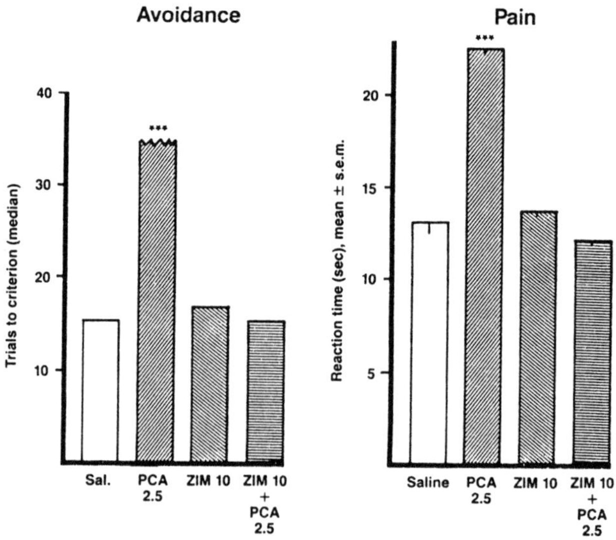

FIGURE 7.3 Zimelidine pretreatment blocks the effects of acute *p*-chloroamphetamine (PCA) treatment on one-way avoidance acquisition and on hot-plate responding in the rat. PCA 2.5 mg/kg was injected 30 min prior to testing and zimelidine (10 mg/kg) 90 min prior to testing. xxx $p < 0.001$ versus saline control. Mann-Whitney U-test, two-tailed.

different location and functional roles these data suggest that release of endogenous 5HT may have different effects on different types of aversive processes.

STUDIES ON THE ROLE OF 5HT NEURONES IN FEAR CONDITIONING AND STRESS-INDUCED ANALGESIA

The active avoidance data do not support the hypothesis that the deficit induced by 5HT release or the alterations in avoidance following 5HT depletion result from similar processes to those involved in nociception. In particular, the observation that different neurochemical mechanisms seem to mediate avoidance and pain is important. However, the interpretation of the active avoidance data is complicated (see Introduction) since the relationship between avoidance performance and shock-level is not linear. This finding led to a series of experiments to examine the involvement of 5HT in shock-induced analgesia and in conditioned fear. It should be pointed out that Watkins and Mayer (1982) have implicated descending pathways in the spinal cord in the inhibition of nociceptive responses by conditioned fear.

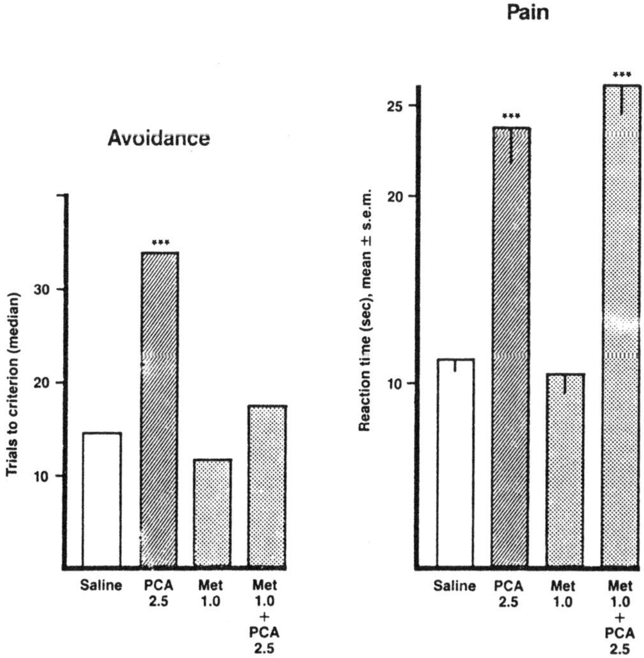

FIGURE 7.4 Metergoline pretreatment blocks the avoidance deficit but not the hot-plate analgesia induced by *p*-chloroamphetamine (PCA) (2.5 mg/kg). Metergoline (MET) was injected 5 min prior to the PCA injection or 35 min before testing. For details, see Figure 7.3 legend.

Previous results from studies on active avoidance indicate that in rats subjected to a prior fear-conditioning procedure, avoidance performance is impaired. This impairment is markedly reduced by *p*-chlorophenylalanine at some shock-levels. In the fear conditioning and fear retention testing procedure (Archer, 1982), each rat is placed in the right-hand compartment of the shuttle-box apparatus used in the active avoidance experiments and 60s later the first of four or eight 2-s shocks (separated by 45s intervals) is delivered. During fear conditioning the gate between the two compartments is always shut. Immediately after the final shock the rat is removed and placed in its home cage. Twenty-four hours later, each rat is placed in the right-hand compartment of the shuttle-box and the gate left open. Latency to locomote and cross over to the non-shock compartment for each rat is recorded.

A number of recent experiments have demonstrated that acute 5HT release produces a marked deficit in fear-retention and passive avoidance retention (Ogren *et al.*, 1981; Archer, 1982). Thus, *p*-chloroamphetamine produces a dose-related deficit in fear-retention when examined 24h after acquisition

(Archer *et al.*, 1981; Archer, 1982). On the other hand, the drug does not appear to block the acquisition of fear (Archer *et al.*, 1981). Pretreatment with zimelidine but not desipramine blocked the retention deficit. A selective role for 5HT in fear retention is further indicated since degeneration of 5HT neurones with *p*-chloroamphetamine (2 × 10 mg/kg) blocked the deficit while long-term treatment with the NA neurotoxin DSP4 (1 × 50 mg/kg), failed to block the acute action of the drug. Interestingly, depletion of 5HT by *p*-chlorophenylalanine (unlike in the previous active avoidance work) did not completely block the fear retention deficit caused by acute *p*-chloroamphetamine (Archer *et al.*, 1982). This finding has been replicated several times.

In another series of experiments we attempted to determine whether the shock-procedure used to produce fear-acquisition also produced shock-induced analgesia. The neurochemical basis for the induced analgesia was also examined. To do this, each animal was examined after inescapable shock at three different shock levels (0.75, 1.25, and 3.0 mA). The rats received either four or eight inescapable shocks at three different shock levels (0.75, 1.25, and 3.0 mA) using the previously described design for fear-conditioning. Three different experiments were performed as follows. Groups of eight rats were injected with either *p*-chloroamphetamine (2 × 10 mg/kg) or saline (2 × 5 mg/kg) 7 and 8 days before fear conditioning, or with *p*-chlorophenylalanine (200, 100, 100 mg/kg) 70, 46, and 22h beforehand. Thirty min before the testing procedure described above, animals from all three groups were injected again with either 2.5 mg/kg *p*-chloroamphetamine or saline. The fear conditioning and retention testing procedure was as described above. The test for analgesia consisted of placing the rat on a hot-plate at 58°C (Ogren and Holm, 1980) and recording the latency to the first observable response (paw-licking or lifting of hind or fore-leg). A pretest value was obtained 10 min prior to the fear-acquisition procedure (T_1). Immediately following the four or eight shocks, the rats were removed from the box and tested for analgesia (T_2). They were also tested 10 and 20 min later (T_3 and T_4). Between each testing each rat was placed in the shock-compartment.

The results for the saline pretreated group are shown in Figure 7.5. In the absence of footshock there was no analgesic response during serial testing following repeated exposure to the avoidance box. Analgesia was dependent both on number and strength of the footshocks. However, it should be noted that in the rats given four shocks, only 3.0 mA produced significant analgesia whereas in those given eight shocks this was observed with both 1.25 and 3.0 mA shock. Thus, in the standard fear-conditioning situation (4 shocks, 1.0 mA) (Archer *et al.*, 1981) shock-induced analgesia probably does not occur.

It can be seen from Figure 7.5 that 30 min after injecting *p*-chloroamphetamine (2.5 mg/kg) to increase 5HT release, response latencies were increased in those animals subsequently exposed to eight shocks at 0.75 and 1.25 mA intensity even before shock onset. It is therefore difficult to determine the

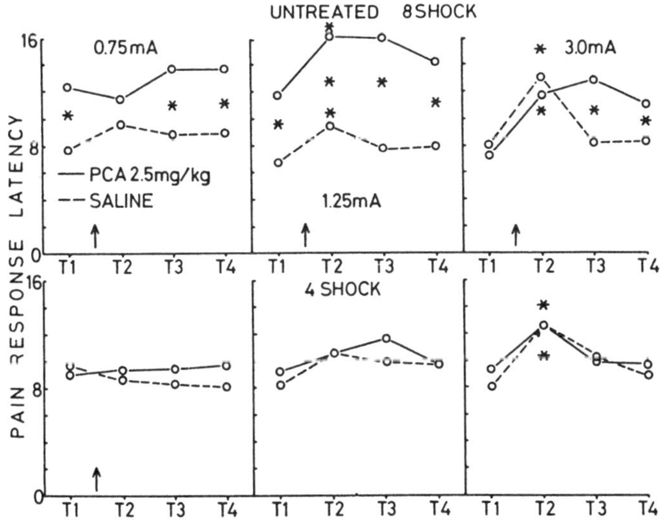

Figure 7.5 Shock-induced analgesia following acute *p*-chloroamphetamine (2.5 mg/kg) in previously untreated rats. Three different shock intensities were used: 0.75, 1.25, and 3.0 mA and either eight shocks (top) or four shocks (bottom). The arrow indicates when shocks were presented. Hot-plate testing of pain response latencies was carried out immediately before and after shock treatment (T_1 and T_2, respectively), 10 min after T_2 (T_3), and 10 min after T_3 (T_4).
$^*p < 0.05$, Mann-Whitney U-test. Asterisk adjacent to a value indicates significant difference from T_1. Asterisk between values indicates significant difference between them.

effect of the drug on shock-induced analgesia under these circumstances. However, in the group subsequently exposed to 3.0 mA shock, when *p*-chloroamphetamine did not significantly alter the pre-shock latency, there was clear evidence of an enhancement of the analgesia. Nevertheless, the drug did not alter the analgesic effect of four shocks at any of the three intensities used.

The results from the rats pretreated with *p*-chlorophenylalanine are presented in Figure 7.6. Essentially identical drug treatment has been found to decrease brain 5HT by about 85% (Ogren *et al.*, 1981). The drug completely blocked the increases in analgesia in all shock conditions (Figure 7.6). Also, the analgesic responses in the four-shock experiment were consistently lower than in the absence of the drug (compare with Figure 7.5) indicating that the nociceptive threshold may be lowered in rats with low brain 5HT. Moreover, *p*-chlorophenylalanine tended to attenuate the analgesic effects of *p*-chloroamphetamine (2.5 mg/kg).

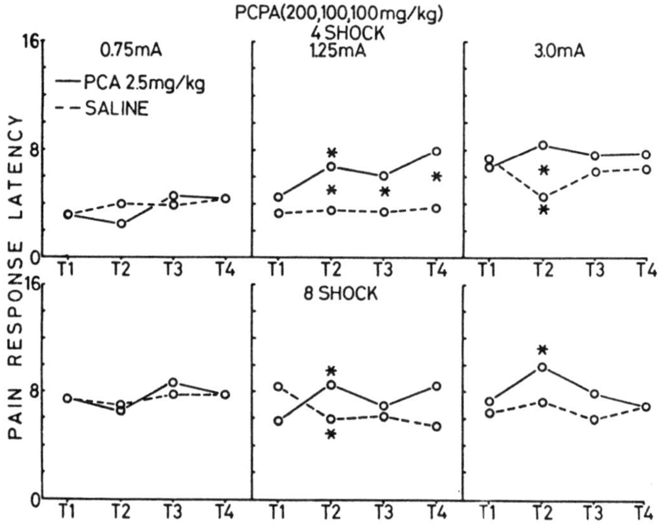

FIGURE 7.6 Shock-induced analgesia following *p*-chloroamphetamine (2.5 mg/kg) in *p*-chlorophenylalanine (PCPA)-treated rats. PCPA (200, 100, 100 mg/kg) was injected 72, 48, and 24h before testing with four shocks (top) or eight shocks (bottom). Significant differences shown as in Figure 7.5.

The results from the rats pretreated with high doses of *p*-chloroamphetamine (2×10 mg/kg) are presented in Figure 7.7. It is evident that this treatment did not change basal levels of analgesia, which is consistent with data obtained from non-stressed animals (Berge *et al.*, 1982). However, it more or less completely blocked the shock-induced analgesia and also attenuated the analgesic effect of acute *p*-chloroamphetamine.

Taken together, these results show that shock-induced analgesia is dependent upon 5HT availability. It is of interest that they are consistent with data obtained using prolonged immobilization stress (Bhattacharya *et al.*, 1978) but not with data obtained by Curzon, Hutson, and Tricklebank who found that acute *p*-chloroamphetamine injection blocks while *p*-chlorophenylalanine enhances analgesia induced by 0.5 min footshock (Tricklebank *et al.*, 1982). However, these authors using both hot-plate and tail-flick procedures and more prolonged shock-treatment have shown attenuation of analgesia by *p*-chlorophenylalanine (Hutson *et al.*, this volume). It is probable, therefore, that procedural differences explain the different results.

These results, as a whole, demonstrate that rats pretreated with *p*-chloroamphetamine, while under training or in the acquisition trial, may have reduced sensitivity or responsiveness to nociceptive stimulation. The changes in nociception appear not to modify fear-acquisition since the animals show the

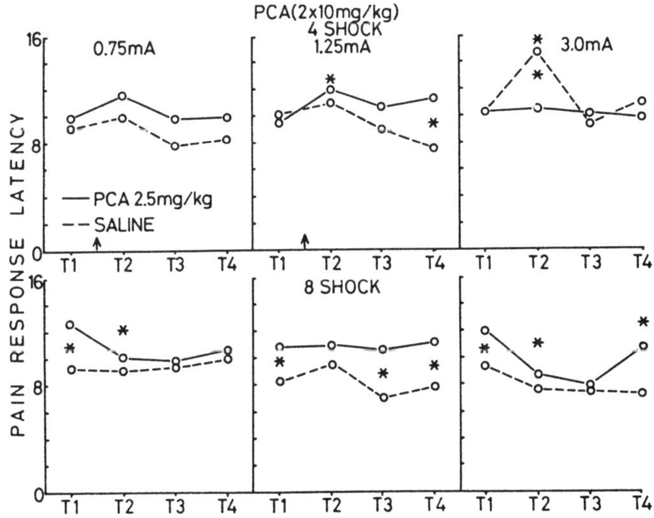

Figure 7.7 Shock-induced analgesia following acute *p*-chloroamphetamine (PCA) (7.5 mg/kg) in PCA-treated rats. PCA (2 × 10 mg/kg) was injected 8 and 7 days before testing with four shocks (top) or eight shocks (bottom). Significant differences shown as in Figure 7.5.

typical immobility of fear-conditioned rats after training. However, when tested 24 h later they show a clear loss of fear retention accompanied by a loss of fear-induced analgesia (to be published). Rats treated with *p*-chlorophenylalanine on the other hand, which tend to show reduced shock-induced analgesia during acquisition, do not display any fear-retention deficit 24 h later. This pretreatment completely blocks the enhancement of analgesia by *p*-chloroamphetamine but does not reduce the 24 h fear-retention deficit (Archer *et al.*, 1982), although the induction of one-way and two-way avoidance deficit by *p*-chloroamphetamine is reduced (Ogren *et al.*, 1981). Depletion of 5HT with high doses of *p*-chloroamphetamine (2 × 10 mg/kg) does not alter shock-induced analgesia but blocks completely the acute effects of this drug on analgesia and on 24 h fear retention deficit. In conclusion, both the fear-conditioning and shock-induced analgesia procedures involve central 5HT and the results as a whole indicate both similarities and differences in their characteristics.

CONCLUSIONS

The present results indicate that aversive learning is not a simple consequence of exposure to aversive stimuli. Thus, the presentation of shock, shock intensity, and whether the shock is escapable or non-escapable have important consequences for avoidance performance. Of particular importance is shock controllability, since pre-exposure to an aversive event, e.g. exposure to shock prior to avoidance learning is detrimental for subsequent performance (Overmier and Seligman, 1976; Jackson *et al.*, 1979). Such a procedure results in acquisition of fear and may influence both stress-induced reaction and associative effects, e.g. the processes which mediate the acquisition of the task. However, it should be noted that avoidance performance cannot be directly related to changes in nociceptive responses. Neither can these results easily be explained in terms of the two-factor theory of avoidance or other current ideas on aversive learning (see Introduction). For instance, changes in nociceptive threshold cannot explain the low avoidance performance by rats treated with *p*-chlorophenylalanine at low and at high shock levels. Moreover, as 5HT depletion blocks shock-induced analgesia, an explanation in terms of nociceptive threshold is not easily applicable. The nature of the underlying mechanisms by which controllable or escapable shock produce changes in nociception and how they relate to avoidance performance is, therefore, unknown. It is possible that there may be different thresholds for elicitation of fear-motivation and pain-inhibition systems and that these thresholds may differ according to the aversive task.

These results also show that acquisition of fear can be achieved without induction of shock-induced analgesia. However, high or repeated shock levels cause shock-induced analgesia and this can be reinstated when animals are re-exposed to a place associated with the shock (to be published). Thus, prolonged shock-exposure activates pain-inhibition systems and the resultant stress-induced analgesia responses may be affected by conditioning. It, is, therefore, of interest that 5HT neurones have been demonstrated to have important roles in avoidance, in escape from aversive shock, in the retention of aversive responses and in the analgesic reactions to shock. However, as there are differences with respect to both encoding and retention between avoidance learning and shock-induced analgesia following 5HT release, 5HT-dependent processes which are involved appear not to be subserved by identical mechanisms. Taken together, both associative and non-associative effects appear to be involved in responses to noxious shock. The relative contribution of conditioning in different aversive learning and shock-induced analgesia paradigms remains to be determined.

REFERENCES

Amir, S., Brown, Z., and Amit, Z. (1980). The role of endorphins in stress: Evidence and speculations. *Neurosci. Biobehav. Rev.*, **4**, 77–86.

Anisman, H., Remington, G., and Sklar, L. (1979). Effects of inescapable shock on subsequent escape performance: catecholaminergic and cholinergic mediation of response initiation and maintenance. *Psychopharmacol.,* **6**, 107–124.

Archer, T. (1982). Serotonin and fear retention in the rat. *J. Comp. Physiol. Psychol.,* **96**, 491–516.

Archer, T., Ogren, S. O., and Johansson, C. (1981). The acute effect of *p*-chloroamphetamine on the retention of fear conditioning in the rat: Evidence for a role of serotonin in memory consolidation. *Neurosic. Letters,* **25**, 75–81.

Archer, T., Ogren, S. O., and Ross, S. B. (1982). Serotonin involvement in aversive conditioning: reversal of the fear retention deficit by long-term *p*-chloroamphetamine but not *p*-chlorophenylalanine. *Neuroscience letters*, **34**, 75–82.

Berge, O.-G. (1982). Effects of 5-HT receptor agonists and antagonists on a reflex response to radiant heat in normal and spinally transected rats. *Pain,* **13**, 253–266.

Berge, O.-G., Hole, K., and Ogren, S. O. (1983). Attenuation of morphine induced analgesia by *p*-chlorophenylalanine and *p*-chloroamphetamine: test-dependent effects and evidence for brainstem 5-hydroxytryptamine involvement. *Brain Res. Reviews*, **271**, 51–64.

Bhattacharya, S. K., Keskary, P. R., and Sandal, A. K. (1978). Immobilization stress induced antinociception in rats: possible role of serotonin and prostaglandins. *Europ. J. Pharmacol.,* **50**, 83–85.

Blair, R., Galina, Z. H., Holmes, L. J., and Amit, Z. (1982). Stress-induced analgesia: a performance deficit or a change in pain responsiveness? *Behav. Neurol. Biology,* **34**, 152–158.

Buckett, W. R. (1981). Pharmacological studies on stimulation-produced analgesia in mice. *Europ. J. Pharmacol.,* **69**, 281–290.

Chance, W. T., White, A. C., Krynock, G. M., and Rosecrans, J. A. (1979). Auto-analgesia: acquisition, blockade and relationship to opiate binding. *Europ. J. Pharmacol.,* **58**, 461–468.

Chance, W. T. (1980). Autoanalgesia: opiate and nonopiate mechanism. *Neurosci. Biobehav. Rev.,* **4**, 55–68.

Curzon, G., Hutson, P. H., and Tricklebank, M. D. (1980). Role of 5-HT in shock induced analgesia. *Br. J. Pharmacol.,* **70**, 44p.

Curzon, G., Hutson, P. H., and Tricklebank, M. D. (1981). Effects of depleting brain and spinal cord 5-HT on footshock induced analgesia. *Br. J. Pharmacol.,* **74**, 218p.

Essman, W. B. (1973). Neuromolecular modulation of experimentally induced retrograde amnesia. *Confinia neurologia,* **35**, 1–122.

Fibiger, H. C., Mertz, P. H., and Campbell, B. A. (1972). The effect of parachlorophenylalanine on aversion thresholds and reactivity to footshock. *Physiol Behav.,* **8**, 259–263.

Fuxe, K., Ögren, S. O., Agnati, L. F., and Jonsson, G. (1978). Further evidence that methergoline is a central 5-hydroxytryptamine receptor blocking agent. *Neurosci. Letters,* **9**, 195–200.

Görlitz, B. D., and Frey, H. H. (1972). Central monoamines and antinociceptive drug action. *Europ. J. Pharmacol.,* **20**, 171–180.

Hayes, R. L., Bennett, G. J., Newlon, P. G., and Mayer, D. J. (1978a). Behavioural and physiological studies of non-narcotic analgesia in the rat elicited by certain environmental stimuli. *Brain Res.,* **155**, 69–90.

Hayes, R. L., Price, D. D., Bennett, G. J., Wilcox, G. L., and Mayer, D. J. (1978b). Differential effects of spinal cord lesions on narcotic and non-narcotic suppression of nociceptive reflexes: further evidence for the physiological multiplicity of pain modulation. *Brain Res.,* **155**, 91–101.

Harvey, J. A., Schlossberg, A. J., and Yunger, L. M. (1974). Effect of *p*-chlorophenylalanine and brain lesions on pain sensitivity and morphine analgesia in the rat. *Adv. Biochem. Psychopharmacol.,* **10**, 233–245.

Hole, K., Fuxe, K., and Jonsson, G. (1976). Behavioural effects of 5,7-dihydroxytryptamine lesions of ascending 5-hydroxytryptamine pathways. *Brain Res.*, **107**, 385–399.

Jackson, R., Maier, S., and Coon, D. (1979). Long-term analgesic effects of inescapable shock and learned helplessness. *Science*, **106**, 91–93.

Koe, B. K., and Weissman, A. (1966). *p*-Chlorophenylalanine: a specific depletor of brain serotonin. *J. Pharmacol. Exp. Ther.*, **154**, 499–516.

Köhler, C., and Lorens, S. (1978). Open field activity and avoidance behaviour following serotonin depletion. A comparison of the effects of parachlorophenylalanine and electrolytic midbrain raphé lesions. *Pharmacol Biochem. Behav.*, **8**, 223–233.

Köhler, C., Ross, S. B., Srebro, B., and Ögren, S. O. (1978). Long-term biochemical and behavioral effects of *p*-chloroamphetamine in the rat. *Ann. NY Acad. Sci.*, **305**, 645–663.

Lewis, J. W., Cannon, J. T., and Liebeskind, J. C. (1980). Opioid and non-opioid mechanisms of stress analgesia. *Science*, **208**, 623–625.

Lorens, S. A. (1978). Some behavioural effects of serotonin depletion depend on method: A comparison of 5,7-dihydroxytryptamine, *p*-chlorophenylalanine, *p*-chloroamphetamine, and electrolytic raphé lesions. *Ann. NY Acad. Sci.*, **305**, 532–555.

Madden, J., Akil, H., Patrick, R. L., and Barchas, J. D. (1977). Stress induces parallel changes in central opioid levels and pain responsiveness in the rat. *Nature*, **265**, 358–360.

Marsden, C. A., Conti, J., Strope, E., Curzon, G. and Adams, R. N. (1979). Monitoring 5-hydroxytryptamine release in the brain of freely moving unanaesthetized rats using *in vivo* voltametry. *Brain Res.*, **171**, 85–99.

Messing, R. B., Phebus, L., Fischer, L. A., and Lytle, L. D. (1975). Analgetic effect of fluoxetine hydrochloride (Lilly 110140) a specific inhibitor of serotonin uptake. *Psychopharmacology Comm.*, **1**, 511–521.

Messing, R. C., Fischer, L. A., Phebus, L, and Lytle, L. D. (1976). Interaction of diet and drugs in the regulation of brain 5-hydroxyindoles and the response to painful electric shock. *Life Sci.*, **18**, 707–714.

Moyer, K. E., and Korn, J. H. (1966). Effect of UCS intensity on the acquisition and extinction of a one-way avoidance response. *Psychonomic Science*, **4**, 121–122.

Mowrer, O. H. (1947). On the dual nature of learning: a reinterpretation of "conditioning" and problem solving. *Harv. Educ. Rev.*, **17**, 102–148.

Ogren, S. O., (1982a). Central serotonin neurons and learning in the rat, in *Biology of Serotonergic Transmission* (ed. N. N. Osborne), pp. 751–763, Wiley & Sons, London.

Ogren, S. O. (1982b). Forebrain serotonin and avoidance learning: behavioural and biochemical studies on the acute effect of *p*-chloroamphetamine on one-way active avoidance learning in the male rat, *Pharmacol. Biochem. Behav.*, **16**, 881–895.

Ogren, S. O., and Holm, A.-C. (1980). Test-specific effects of the 5-HT reuptake inhibitors alaproclate and zimelidine on pain sensitivity and morphine analgesia. *J. Neural. Transmission*, **47**, 253–271.

Ogren, S. O., and Berge, O. G. (1984). Test dependent variation in the anti-nociceptive effect of parachloroamphetamine induced release of 5-hydroxytryptamine. *Neuropharmacology*, (in press).

Ogren, S. O., and Johansson, C. (1984). Separation of the associative and non-associative effects of parachloroamphetamine induced brain serotonin release. Dissociation between serotonergic involvement in arousal, learning, pain and motor function. *Psychopharmacology*, (submitted).

Ogren, S. O., Ross, S. B., Holm, A.-C., and Baumann, L. (1977). 5-Hydroxytryptamine and avoidance performance in the rat. Antagonism of the acute effect of *p*-chloroamphetamine by zimelidine, an inhibitor of 5-hydroxytryptamine uptake. *Neurosci. Lett.*, **7**, 331–336.

Ogren, S.-O., Fuxe, K., Archer, T., Hall, H., Holm, A.-C., and Köhler, C. (1981). Studies on the role of central 5-HT neurons in avoidance learning: a behavioural and biochemical analysis, in *Serotonin: Current Aspects of Neurochemistry and Function* (eds B. Haber, S. Gabay, M. R. Issidores and S. G. A. Alivisatos), pp. 681–705, Plenum Press, New York.

Ogren, S. O., Johansson, C., Johansson, G., and Archer, T. (1982), Serotonin neurons and aversive conditioning in the rat, *Scand J. Psychol.*, **51**, 7–15.

Overmier, J., and Seligman, M. (1976). Effects of inescapable shock upon subsequent escape and avoidance responding. *J. Comp. Phys. Psychol.*, **63**, 28–33.

Peroutka, S. J., Lebovitz, R. M., and Snyder, S. H. (1981). Two distinct central serotonin receptors with different physiological functions. *Science,* **212**, 827–828.

Rescorla, R., and Solomon, R. (1967). Two process learning theory: Relationships between Pavlovian conditioning and instrumental learning. *Psychol. Rev.*, **74**, 151–182.

Ross, S. B., (1976). Antagonism of the acute and long-term biochemical effects of 4-chloroamphetamine on the 5-HT neurons in the rat brain by inhibitors of the 5-hydroxytryptamine uptake. *Acta Pharmacol. Toxicol.*, **39**, 456–476.

Sanders-Bush , E., and Steranka, L. R. (1978). Immediate and long-term effects of *p*-chloroamphetamine on brain amines. *Ann. NY Acad. Sci.*, **305**, 208–221.

Sastry, B. S. R., and Phillis, J. W. (1977). Metergoline as a selective 5-hydroxytryptamine antagonist in the cerebral cortex. *Can. J. Physiol. Pharmacol.*, **55**, 130–133.

Sewell, R. D. E., and Spencer, P. S. J. (1975). Anti-nociceptive activity of narcotic agonists and partial agonists in mice given biogenic amines by intracerebroventricular injection. *Psychoparmacology,* **42**, 67–71.

Tenen, S. S. (1967). The effects of *p*-chlorophenylalanine, a serotonin depletor on avoidance acquisition, pain sensitivity and behaviour in the rat. *Psychopharmacologia,* **10**, 204–219.

Tricklebank, M. D., Drewitt, P. N., and Curzon, G. (1980). The effect of L-tryptophan on motor activity and its prevention by an extracerebral decarboxylase inhibitor and by 5HT receptor blockers. *Psychopharmacology,* **69**, 173–177.

Tricklebank, M. D., Hutson, P. H., and Curzon, G, (1982). Analgesia induced by brief footshock is inhibited by 5-hydroxytryptamine but unaffected by antagonists of 5-hydroxytryptamine or by naloxone, *Neuropharmacology*, **21** 51–56.

Watkins, L. R., and Mayer, D. J. (1982). Organization of endogenous opiate and nonopiate pain control systems. *Science,* **216**, 1185–1192.

Weiss, J., Glazer, H., Pohorecky, L., Brick, J., and Miller, N. (1975). Effects of chronic exposure to stressors on avoidance-escape behaviour and on brain norepinephrine. *Psychosomatic Medicine,* **37**, 522–534.

Vogt, M. (1974). The effect of lowering the 5-hydroxytryptamine content of the rat spinal cord on analgesia produced by morphine. *J. Physiol.*, **236**, 483–498.

Yaksh, T. L., and Wilson, P. R. (1979). Spinal serotonin terminal system mediates antinociception. *J. Pharmac. Exp. Ther.*, **208**, 446–453.

Stress-induced Analgesia
Edited by M. D. Tricklebank and G. Curzon

CHAPTER 8

Methodological considerations in experiments on stress-induced analgesia

M. D. TRICKLEBANK and G. CURZON

The foregoing chapters leave us in no doubt that an animal's responsiveness to painful stimulation can be modified by environmental stimuli. However, from the original hypothesis that endogenous mechanisms of analgesia exist and are activated when the awareness of pain might impede survival, few would have anticipated the apparent abundance and independence of the mechanisms involved.

Much of the early work in this area was directed towards demonstrating a physiological role for the endogenous opioids. That this has now been achieved is indicated by the antagonism by naloxone of the decrease in responsiveness after stress and the demonstration of cross tolerance between repeatedly-stressed and chronically morphine treated rats. Experimental design has proved crucial to this demonstration, and early negative results can now be explained by the differential activation of opioid and non-opioid dependent pain inhibitory mechanisms.

The importance of stress duration in eliciting naloxone sensitive and insensitive analgesia, first demonstrated by Lewis *et al.* (1980), became less clear when it was subsequently shown that dependency on stress duration depends on the body region to which the insult is applied. Thus, prolonged (20 min), but not acute (3 min) footshock produces a naloxone sensitive analgesia (Lewis *et al.*, 1980) but a shock duration of only 1.5 min is sufficient if the application of shock is restricted to the forepaws (Watkins *et al.*, 1982a).

These results raise the question as to whether opiate sensitive analgesia always involves activation of the same mechanisms. Reported differential sensitivities to hormonal influences could be interpreted to indicate that this is not the case. Thus, if we consider the analgesia induced by brief shock to the forepaws, by prolonged shock, or by brief re-exposure to shock 24h after prolonged shock, we find all three are naloxone sensitive. Nevertheless, the first paradigm is reported to be independent of pituitary-adrenal influences (Watkins *et al.*, 1982b), the second is sensitive to adreno-medullary, but not adrenocortical factors (Lewis *et al.*, 1982), while the third is sensitive only to adrenocortical factors (MacLennon *et al.*, 1982).

It might, however, be prudent to also consider these results as possible indications of the importance of experimental design. The following discussion concerns seven variables or group of variables that can be manipulated independently of one another in the induction of analgesia by stress. In this final chapter, we shall attempt to illustrate the importance of these variables and, with the benefit of hindsight, suggest some design guidelines which might be useful to follow in future studies of stress-induced analgesia.

1. TEST OF NOCICEPTION

The efficacy of even drug-induced analgesia can vary quite markedly with the method of analgesic assessment (Dennis and Melzack, 1980; Ogren and Holm 1980). This is perhaps not too surprising if noxious levels of different physical stimuli that are likely to activate different nociceptive systems are used as the probing stimulus. However, conflicting results can be obtained when different responses to the same stimulus are monitored (Dennis and Melzack, 1980). Stress-induced analgesia is no exception. Thus, in a study using restraint stress, a naloxone sensitive increase in hot plate escape latency, not contingent on non-specific motor effects of the stress, was seen. However, this apparent analgesic effect was not reflected in an increase in the latency to lick the paws (Amir and Amit, 1978). If this had been the sole criterion used (as is often the case) the stress would not have been considered to be analgesic.

2. USE OF PRE-STRESS NOCICEPTIVE TESTING

The increase in tail-flick latency following 30 s footshock only occurred when pre-shock latencies were determined before the shock (Tricklebank *et al.*, 1984). The pharmacology of the phenomenon, which may be more analogous to passive-avoidance behaviour than to stress-induced analgesia, is strikingly different to that seen when shock duration is increased to 30 min, when dependency on pre-shock nociceptive testing is no longer apparent. Many workers incorporate pre-stress determinations of responsiveness in their experimental design, often without specifying the interval between the last determination and exposure to the stress. It is therefore possible that, in some cases, the resultant analgesic response reflects more than one mechanism and that its pharmacology might, as a result, be difficult to interpret.

3. TYPE OF STRESS AND ITS SITE OF APPLICATION

The types of stress which induce analgesia have already been considered in some detail (Bodnar, Chapter 2). It is perhaps worth noting again that not all stressors (defined as manipulations that activate the pituitary–adrenal axis) induce analgesia (Hayes *et al.*, 1978). Stressors vary in their ability to activate nociceptors and have varying degrees of relevance to normal behaviour of the species to which they are applied. For example, the injection of 2-deoxyglucose is unlikely to have the same affective significance for a rat as the presence of an unfamiliar animal, and while both procedures lead to analgesia, the mechanisms by which this is achieved may not be identical. As already mentioned in Section 1 of this chapter the body region to which the stress is applied must also be considered. Electric shock induces analgesia whether applied to the forepaws, to all paws or only to the hindpaws but only the analgesia induced by forepaw shock is reported to be blocked by naloxone (Watkins *et al.*, 1982a).

4. INTENSITY, FREQUENCY, AND DURATION OF STRESS

The importance of stress duration has been commented on above and also in Chapter 5 by Lewis *et al*. The possibility that different intensities or frequencies of stress can activate different analgesic mechanisms has not yet been systematically investigated, but remains a possibility.

5. TIME BETWEEN TERMINATION OF STRESS AND POST-STRESS NOCICEPTIVE TESTING

Analgesia can be detected in animals immediately on termination of brief footshock and usually has a duration of 15–20 min. The immediate post-stress effect often appears relatively resistant to pharmacological antagonism. This has been demonstrated for antagonism by naloxone (Watkins *et al.*, 1982a) and by monoamine receptor antagonists (Snow *et al.*, 1982). It could indicate that these drugs affect the decay of the analgesic response rather than its induction or that the mechanism of the initial analgesia effect is different from that of the analgesia which is detectable later.

6. DURATION AND FREQUENCY OF POST-STRESS NOCICEPTIVE TESTING

Repeated exposure of animals to the nociceptive test is an important variable in the development of analgesic tolerance to morphine (Advocat and Isaac, 1983). The decay of the analgesic response to stress might be similarly accelerated by repeated testing though this remains to be demonstrated. One situation in which repeated post-shock testing may conceivably affect analgesic responses is when this depends on pre-stress nociceptive testing (see Section 2 of this chapter) as subsequent analgesia tests, not followed by the imposition of stress, might obliterate any association made between test and stress.

7. USE OF BRIEF RE-EXPOSURE TO STRESS BEFORE NOCICEPTIVE TESTING

The 'reinduction' of analgesia by brief re-exposure to footshock some time after a prolonged period of shock has design analogies with experiments demonstrating learned helplessness. This procedure has been claimed to induce a purer form of opioid-mediated analgesia, uninfluenced by the motor deficits possibly present immediately after prolonged shock (MacLennon *et al.*, 1982). However, such experiments may involve numerous uncertainties related to learning and memory, and thus be difficult to interpret with confidence.

COMMENT

It is not surprising that studies of the mechanisms of stress-induced analgesia have produced so many seemingly conflicting results. An important task for the future is to detect those factors that are of secondary importance (interesting though they may often be), in the hope that this will allow the development of standardized model analgesia systems that can be more easily interpreted. Confusion might be avoided if for example, the tests of analgesia were restricted to the simpler nociceptive reflexes and if the post-stress analgesia was shown to be either dependent or independent of pre-stress nociceptive testing or an association with any other pre-stress experience. Under these circumstances, assessment of the importance of such factors as duration, frequency, and intensity of stress may prove to be an easier task. Unfortunately it is not always easy to quantitatively assess and systematically vary stress intensity. However, with modern telemetric techniques it might be possible to monitor other physiological effects of the stress, such as changes in the EEG, heart rate, and blood pressure. Also, blood might be sampled via indwelling catheters and used to determine plasma catecholamines and corticosteroids. Knowledge of these parameters would help in assessing the significance of the stress to the animal. As Devor points out (Chapter 1) such knowledge might help to explain why seemingly minor changes in experimental protocol can result in the activation of apparently different analgesic mechanisms.

Finally, we should, nevertheless, acknowledge that the sensitivity of stress-induced analgesia to experimental design has already led to important insights into factors influencing endogenous analgesic mechanisms. The present comments on experimental design do not detract from the substantial progress already made. It is hoped, however, that they will help the interpretation of existing data and the development of future research.

REFERENCES

Advocat, C., and Isaac, L. (1983). Nociceptive assessment modifies behavioural tolerance without altering brain morphine concentration. *Europ. J. Pharmacol.*, **92**, 135–138.

Amir, S., and Amit, Z. (1978). Endogenous opioid ligands may mediate stress-induced changes in the affective properties of pain related behaviour in rats. *Life Sci.,* **23**, 1143–1152.

Dennis, S. G., and Melzack, R. (1980). Pain modulations by 5-hydroxytryptamine agents and morphine as measured by three pain tests. *Expt. Neurol.,* **69**, 260–270.

Hayes, R. L., Bennett, G. J., Newlon, P. G., and Mayer, D. J. (1978). Behavioural and physiological studies of non-narcotic analgesia in the rat elicited by certain environmental stimuli. *Brain Res.,* **155**, 69–90.

Lewis, J. W., Cannon, J. T., and Liebeskind, J. C. (1980). Opioid and non-opioid mechanisms of stress analgesia. *Science,* **208**, 623–625.

Lewis, J. W., Tordoff, M. G., Sherman, J. E., and Liebeskind, J. C. (1982). Adrenal medullary enkephalin-like peptides may mediate opioid stress analgesia. *Science,* **217**, 557–559.

MacLennon, A. J., Drugan, R. C., Hyson, R. L., Maier, S. F., Madden, J., and Barchas, J. D. (1982). Corticosterone: a critical factor in an opioid form of stress-induced analgesia. *Science,* **215**, 1530–1532.

Ogren, S. O., and Holm, A.-C. (1980). Test specific effects of the 5HT reuptake inhibitors alaproclate and zimelidine on pain sensitivity and morphine analgesia. *J. Neural. transmission,* **47**, 253–271.

Snow, A. E., Tucker, S. M., and Dewey, W. L. (1982). The role of neurotransmitters in stress-induced antinociception (SIA). *Pharmac. Biochem. Behav.,* **16**, 47–50.

Tricklebank, M. D., Hutson P. H., and Curzon G. (1984). Analgesia induced by brief or more prolonged stress differs in its dependency on naloxone, 5-hydroxytryptamine and previous analgesia testing. *Neuropharmacology,* **23**, 417–421.

Watkins, L. R., Cobelli, D. A., Faris, P., Aceto, M. D., and Meyer, D. J. (1982a). Opiate vs non-opiate footshock-induced analgesia (FSIA): The body region shocked is a critical factor. *Brain Res.,* **242**, 299–308.

Watkins, L. R., Cobelli, D. A., Newsome, H. H., and Mayer, D. J. (1982b). Footshock induced analgesia is dependent neither on pituitary nor sympathetic activation. *Brain Res.,* **245**, 81–96.

Index